SIRTFOOD DIET

The Original SirtFood Diet Cookbook to Lose Weight and Gain Health with No Sacrifices by Activating the Skinny Gene While Eating Chocolate and Drinking Wine

© Copyright 2019 by Adam Goggins
All rights reserved.

This document is geared towards providing exact and reliable information with regards to the topic and issue covered. The publication is sold with the idea that the publisher is not required to render accounting, officially permitted, or otherwise, qualified services. If advice is necessary, legal or professional, a practiced individual in the profession should be ordered.

- From a Declaration of Principles which was accepted and approved equally by a Committee of the American Bar Association and a Committee of Publishers and Associations.

In no way is it legal to reproduce, duplicate, or transmit any part of this document in either electronic means or in printed format. Recording of this publication is strictly prohibited and any storage of this document is not allowed unless with written permission from the publisher. All rights reserved.

The information provided herein is stated to be truthful and consistent, in that any liability, in terms of inattention or otherwise, by any usage or abuse of any policies, processes, or directions contained within is the solitary and utter responsibility of the recipient reader. Under no circumstances will any legal responsibility or blame be held against the publisher for any reparation, damages, or monetary loss due to the information herein, either directly or indirectly.

Respective authors own all copyrights not held by the publisher.

The information herein is offered for informational purposes solely, and is universal as so. The presentation of the information is without contract or any type of guarantee assurance.

The trademarks that are used are without any consent, and the publication of the trademark is without permission or backing by the trademark owner. All trademarks and brands within this book are for clarifying purposes only and are the owned by the owners themselves, not affiliated with this document

Table of Contents

Chapter 1: The Science of Sirtuins 1
- Of Mince and Men 1
- An Appetite for Fasting? 2
- A Zeal for Exercise? 4
- Enter Sirtfoods 5

Chapter 2: Sirtfoods Explained 7
- What are SIRTs? 7
- What do SIRTs do? 7
- Food Safety Mistakes 9
- Pros and Cons: 16

Chapter 3: Best Sirtfoods 18
- Food Names 18
- Diet Boosting Foods 38

Chapter 4: How to Build Muscles 44
- Sirtuins and Muscles Mass 45
- Sirtfoods VS Fasting 46
- Keeping Muscles Young 47

Chapter 5: Build a Diet That Works 51
- Tips to build the sirtfood diet that better fits for you 51
- Hitting Your Quota 52
- The Power of Synergy 53
- Juicing and Food: Get the Best of Both Worlds 55
- The Power of Protein 57
- Eat Early 59
- Go Big on Taste 61
- Embrace Eating 63
- What to Expect 68
- How to Follow Phase 1 69

Phase 2: Maintenance 81
- What to Expect 81
- How to Follow Phase 2 82

After the Diet 92

Chapter 6: Sirtfood Recipes 94
- Asian Shrimp Stir-Fry with Buckwheat Noodles 96
- Miso and Sesame Glazed Tofu with Ginger and Chili Stir-Fried Greens 98
- Turkey Escalope with Sage, Capers, Parsley and Spiced Cauliflower Couscous 101
- Kale and Red Onion Dal with Buckwheat 103
- Aromatic Chicken Breast with Kale Red Onions, and Tomato and Chili Salsa 105
- HARISSA BAKED TOFU WITH CAULIFLOWER "COUSCOUS" 107
- Sirt Muesli 109
- Pan-Fried Salmon Fillet With Caramelized Endive, Arugula, and Cherry Leaf Salad 111
- Tuscan Bean Stew 113
- Strawberry Buckwheat Tabbouleh 115
- Miso-Marinated Baked Cod with Stir-Fried Greens and Sesame 116
- Soba (Buckwheat Noodles) in a Miso Broth with Tofu, Celery, and Kale 118
- Sirt Super Salad 120
- Char-Grilled Beef with a Red Wine Jus, Onion Rings, Garlic Kale, and Herb-Roasted Potatoes 122
- Steak Cooking Times 125
- Kidney Bean Mole with Baked Potato 126
- Sirtfood Omelet 128
- Baked Chicken Breast with Walnut and Parsley Pesto and Red Onion Salad 130
- Waldorf Salad 132
- Roasted Eggplant Wedges with Walnut and Parsley Pesto and Tomato Salad 134
- Sirtfood Smoothie 136
- Stuffed Whole-Wheat Pita 137
- Butternut Squash and Date Tagine with Buckwheat 139
- Butter Bean and Miso Dip With Celery Sticks and

Oatcakes 141
Yogurt with Berries, Walnuts, and Dark Chocolate 143
Chicken And Kale Curry With Bombay Potatoes 144
Spiced Scrambled Eggs 147
Sirt Chili Con Carne 148
Mushroom and Tofu Scramble 150
Smoked Salmon Pasta with Chili and Arugula 152
Buckwheat Pasta Salad 154
Buckwheat Pancakes with Strawberries, Dark Chocolate Sauce, and Squeezed Walnuts 155
Tofu and Shiitake Mushroom Soup 158
Sirtfood Bites 160
Quinoa, Chickpea and Turmeric Curry 162
Savory Turmeric Pancakes with Lemon Yogurt Sauce .. 164
Blueberry Smoothie 167
Blueberry Banana Pancakes with Chunky Apple Compote and Golden Turmeric Latte 168
Buckwheat Superfood Muesli 171
Mocha Chocolate Mousse 173
Moroccan Spiced Eggs 176
Vietnamese Turmeric Fish with Herbs & Mango Sauce 178
Sirtfood Diet's Shakshuka 182
Sirtfood Diet's Braised Puy Lentils 184
Salmon Sirt Super Salad 186
Chinese-Style Pork with Pak Choi 188

Chapter 7: How to Lose Fat 190
List of Sirtuin activating, fat burning SIRTfoods 190

Chapter 8: Maintain a healthy life 193
Doing exercise with the diet 193
Sirtfood diet during pregnancy 194
Sirtfood diet for children 195
Sirtfood diet for people on medication 195
Cancer Prevention Foods 196

Chapter 1
The Science of Sirtuins

The sirfood diet is based on research on SIRTs or sirtuins. These are a group of seven proteins found in the human body that regulate functions like metabolism, inflammation, and lifespan, according to a study. The sirtfood diet works on the assumption that certain plant compounds may be able to increase level of these proteins. These plants are dubbed as sirtfoods.

A combination of sirtfoods along with calorie restriction could trigger the body to produce higher levels of sirtuins, leading to rapid weight loss, while maintaining muscle mass.

Of Mince and Men

In recent times, sirtuins have, unsurprisingly, become the focus of extensive science investigation. The first sirtuin was detected in yeast back in 1984, and research really began over the span of the next 30 years when it was realized that sirtuin stimulation enhances life span, first in yeast and then all the way to the top to mice.

Why the thrills? Because from yeast to humans and everything else in between, the basic values of cell metabolic processes are remarkably similar. If you can control anything as small as a burgeoning yeast to see a gain and replicate it in higher species like mice, there is hope for the same advantages to be discovered in humans.

An Appetite for Fasting?

That also helps to bring us to fasting. Continuously, the lifetime reduction of food consumption has been found to increase the life span of lower species and mammals. This awesome finding is the foundation for the exercise of caloric restriction among certain people, where regular calorie intake is decreased by around twenty to thirty percent, as well as its helped popularize offshoot, irregular fasting, that has become an effective weight-loss nutrition, partly inspired by the likes of the 5:2 diet, or Fast Diet. While we're still waiting for evidence of increased lifetime for human beings from these procedures, there's evidence of advantages to what we might call "health period"—chronic disease drops, and fat falls down away.

But let's be truthful. No matter how large the advantages, dieting week in, and week out is an exhausting business that many of us don't want to sign up for. Even when we do, most of us are not prepared to adhere to this. Besides this there are disadvantages to fasting, particularly if we follow it for a long time. We listed in the intro the adverse effects of hunger, tiredness, weakness, muscular failure and slowing in metabolic rate. But continuing fasting schemes could also put us at risk of food insecurity, impacting our health-being due to a reduced availability of fats nutrients. Fasting systems are often entirely inadequate for vast numbers of the population such as infants, females during gestation, and most likely older people. Although fasting has obviously proven advantages, it's not the silver bullet we 'd want it to be. It had us question whether this was the way Nature was meant to make us thin, fit, and active? There's obviously a good way out there.

Our discovery came when we learned that our old sirtuin genes were enabled by mediating the substantial advantages from caloric restriction and abstinence. Thinking of sirtuins as the defenders at the intersection of energy status and immortality may be beneficial to fully understand this. There, what they do is react to stress and strain.

When energy is in limited supply, there is a rise in tension on our cells just as we see in the calorie limit. The sirtuins detected this, and then turned on and transmitted a series of potent signals that dramatically altered the behavior of cells. Sirtuins start increasing our metabolism, increase our muscular productivity, switch on fat loss, reducing pain and fix the damage in our cells. Sirtuins, in turn, make us fit and healthy, slimmer, and safer.

There are 7 distinct sirtuins in humans (SIRT1 to SIRT7). Of these, the single most significant sirtuins associated with energy equilibrium are SIRT1 and SIRT3. Although SIRT1 is present in the body, SIRT3 is located mainly in our mitochondria—the cells' energy-main house. Their stimulation next to each other gives us the many advantages that we are hoping to achieve.

A Zeal for Exercise?

It isn't just caloric limitation and fasting that triggers sirtuins; exercise also does. As in fasting, sirtuins organize the profound advantages of workout. Yet while we are urged to participate in routine, physical activity for its myriad of advantages, it is not the mechanism on which we are expected to concentrate our attention on weight-loss. Evidence indicates that the human body has developed ways of adapting spontaneously and that the energy and power that we consume while exercising, which ensures that in order for fitness to be a successful weight-loss strategy, we have to devote lots of time and effort. The grueling fitness regimens are the way evolution designed us to sustain a healthier weight seems much more questionable in the face of studies now showing that exercising too much may be dangerous to undermine our immune systems, damage the heart and lead to early mortality.

Enter Sirtfoods

So far, we have realized that the key to activating our sirtuin genes is if we want to lose some weight and be healthful. Fasting and meditation have been the 2 main ways of doing that up to now. Unfortunately, the sums required for good weight loss come with their disadvantages, but for most of us, this is clearly inconsistent with how we lead 21st century lives. Luckily, there is a recently found, ground-breaking way to activate our sirtuin genes in the effective manner possible: sirtfood. As we will soon discover, these are the miracle foods that are especially abundant in unique plant-natural chemicals, which have the capacity to converse with our sirtuin genes and turn them on. In fact, they imitate the impact of abstinence and workout and in doing so, offer incredible advantages of losing weight, muscle strengthening, and health improving that were formerly unachievable.

SUMMARY

- We each have an ancestral gene group, called sirtuins.
- Primary metabolic controllers are sirtuins that regulate our capacity to lose fat and remain alive.
- Sirtuins serve as energy detectors in our cells and are triggered when energy deficits are observed.
- Fasting and workout both stimulate our sirtuin

genes but may be difficult to adhere to and may even have disadvantages.
- Our sirtuin genes are being programmed in a new innovative way: sirtfoods.
- You can counteract the action of fasting and workout by eating a diet that is rich in Sirtfoods and accomplish the body you desire.

Chapter 2
Sirtfoods Explained

What are SIRTs?

SIRTs, or sirtuins, are a group of enzymes that control key biological cell growth reactions. Owing to their ability to improve fat loss, super increasing your activity levels, and perhaps even prolonging your life, their invention has created tremendous anticipation.

The very first SIRT was identified in yeast cells and assigned SIR2 (Silent Information Regulator 2) protein, a very unexceptional name. These were pointed to as SIRTs or sirtuins as related proteins were eventually discovered in human cells. 7 human SIRT proteins have been found already and have been titled SIRT1 to SIRT7.

What do SIRTs do?

Sirtuin proteins are enzymes that have a critical part to

play in how cells adapt to meals, exercise as well as other influences in lifestyles. SIRTs operate with the cells, fine-tuning their output so that each cell works much effectively. They achieve so by modifying different proteins and fatty acids present in the cell nuclei, cell liquid (cytoplasm) and energy-producing cell components (mitochondria) into the chemical composition.

This specific alteration inside the nucleus (the most important of which is a synthetic snip known as diacylation) leads to activation or inhibition of cell genes involved. Such gene modifications, combined, allow the cells to:

- Turbocharging generates cellular capacity
- Boost reducing fat
- Facilitating favorable weight loss
- Trigger channels for cell protection to reduce inflammation
- DNA harmed in repair
- Regrow worn out components of cells (organelles)
- Lengthen the cell viability during stressful periods due to factors such as lack of oxygen, disease, or pathogen build-up
- Place new synaptic connections within the brain to facilitate memory development, preservation, and recovery.

Each sirtuin protein is focused according to function inside particular parts of each cell.

SIRT1, SIRT6, and SIRT7 are found primarily in the cell nucleus and are involved in the regulation how genes are managed to switch on and off in reply to certain stimuli – including all those genes responsible for the SIRT proteins themselves. SIRT7 has been mostly focused mainly inside of the nuclear membrane in an area known as the nucleolus, where protein-making apparatus of the cell is controlled.

SIRT2 is predominantly found in cell plasma (cytoplasm) where it controls cellular metabolism and also has cell regeneration and DNA repair associated anti-ageing activities.

SIRT3, SIRT4, and SIRT5 are found primarily inside the mitochondria – the relatively small, ever-ready devices that produce energy in each cell. SIRT3 is intimately correlated to the process of aging and long life while SIRT4 has particular insulin sensitivity-related actions.

Food Safety Mistakes

1. Transporting Groceries from the Store to Home

One basic principle is to keep foods frozen or refrigerated at all times. Even at a slow pace, microbes will grow rapidly in your food once they start to warm up.

If it takes you more than 30 minutes to get to your home from the grocery store, plan ahead and keep a cooler inside your car. And if you're planning to go to the grocery store, make sure you've got that cooler ready to go (with an ice pack!) and ideally last stop at the grocery store (and last shop during your food trip).

If you're not using a cooler but go straight home, keep the perishable foods in front of your car where there is air conditioning and it's cooler as a result. Keep in mind that perishables can only be kept in a cooler till microbes start to develop for around two hours.

2. Properly Reheating Leftovers

Leftover food is always a great option, especially if you're crunched for time, but did you know that not properly heating the leftovers is a major cause of foodborne disease?

First and foremost: Ensure that the leftovers are refrigerated properly when putting them away. Many people assume that leftovers need to be cooled before cooling, but that actually increases microbe's development, so get them in the fridge ASAP (or at least within 2 hours).

Second: Take your food to at least 165 degrees F or until the food is steaming (if you are super vigilant you can use a food thermometer for double checking). Using microwaves to heat up leftovers is very common, although not always consistent when heating food through, so double check that your entire entry is hot before consuming.

3. Cross Contamination

Cross contamination is currently the leading cause of foodborne disease people think of (think cooked; the meat of BBQ is put back in same dish in which it was marinated). It's also one of the easiest food safety errors to fix with a little attention to detail.

So long as you distinguish ready-to-eat foods from raw meats & clean utensils or materials that may have come into contact with raw meats, you're more likely in the clear. Do not hesitate to get your cutting boards washed! (Wash them in wet, soapy water and if you really want to keep them clean, spritz or rinse them with white vinegar. You can place them in dishwasher to sanitize if you use a plastic cutting board).

These safety measures are extremely significant, since raw meat bacteria are extremely easy to transfer.

4. Thawing Frozen Foods

Everybody has a way they've been learned to thaw frozen foods, but actually there was a right or wrong way to do it ... but most of us are messing that up.

Actually, only 62 percent of people thaw their frozen foods correctly. Frozen foods must be defrosted N-O-T on the countertop because the food can attain a temperature between 40-140 degrees F which is the term "the danger zone" for food safety experts. This maximum temperature is where pathogens multiply most rapidly. Even if you don't think this is risky, it is.

The finest (and safest) way to thaw your frozen food is through your refrigerator. This helps the frozen item to thaw gradually without going into "the danger zone." if that isn't possible, like failing to thaw your steak for dinner, you can defrost frozen food in a big bowl of cool water (just make sure it's in an airtight box or plastic bag – and don't forget it overnight on the counter!).

5. Not Washing Your Hands (or not washing them properly)

This one looks simple but could very easily get you sick. Wash your hands after handling, when working with raw poultry, meat, fish or eggs.

Which means BEFORE you touch anything – tongs, saltshakers or even a kitchen towel, when your hands are not very well cleaned, pathogens expand to EVERYTHING that you contact. And no, not putting your hands under water counts.

To reduce pathogen spread, you should wash your hands with soap and warm water. Most people don't wash their hands almost as thoroughly (or as frequently as they should). A rule of thumb is to wash your hands for as long as reciting the ABC's takes you. This may sound a little (or very) dumb, but it guarantees you don't spread bacteria in your kitchen.

6. Using Raw Meat Marinade on Cooked Meat

The last thing you want to think about when relaxing at a BBQ is food poisoning.

While marinating your meat before cooking is a good practice (see why this post is about), you should NOT use the marinade with which raw meat has come into contact. Go for a fresh marinade batch as a sauce or boil it first to destroy any nasty pathogens.

7. Not Replacing (or Sanitizing) Sponges and Dishrags

Cross-contamination is super normal as discussed above, but have you ever thought about all the bacteria harboring in your sponge and dish rags you pass all the time?

Like cutting boards, sponges and dishrags are porous which make them a breeding ground for pathogens and germs. This is best to sanitize sponges every other day to avoid this (you can soak them in white vinegar, run them through the dishwasher, or nuke them in the microwave (when wet!) for 60 seconds on "high") and sometimes replace them.

(And please don't use the dishwashing sponges to wipe down your counters! That commits mistake #3!)

Make it a routine to wash your kitchen towels 2-3x a week (ideally in HOT water) or more frequently as needed. This will make sure that pathogens don't spread around your kitchen.

8. Washing Poultry Before Preparing

Raw poultry is one of the food products which is most often polluted. Perhaps that's why some people get used to "cleaning" it by rinsing it in the sink before cooking, but it's currently been shown to expand bacteria around the kitchen. Chicken water droplets (even the small ones you can't see) are a possible source of pollution.

In particular, any surface it touches should be disinfected when preparing poultry-or any meat for that matter. But cleaning the meat increases the region that needs disinfection. Unfortunately, we are not superhuman, so when washed, we cannot see every place the poultry touches.

If food safety is essential to you, it is better not to wash the poultry before preparing it and instead ensure that you cook it at the proper temperature to kill any pathogens (165 degrees F).

9. Assuming Raw Vegetables are Safe

This could be the biggest misconception people have concerning food safety.

Many of us believe we can only get sick from raw meat, but did you know that salmonella can be harbored by a cantaloupe's rind? Or that leafy greens often become contaminated with E. coli?

Fresh produce accounts for almost half of the foodborne illnesses, so in reality it is very important to properly prepare and store the produce. Ensure that perishable products are kept in a refrigerator in a crisper drawer and are not handled with dirty hands. Rinse your produce before feeding (use a diluted mixture of vinegar-water to help reduce surface bacteria). Buying local farmers' produce decreases the risk of food poisoning, as many of the products responsible for major outbreaks have been related to contamination in giant processing plants.

10. Separation of Food in the Fridge

Most people would put food anywhere they can find room in their refrigerator, but in reality, there is a proper way to place food to avoid contamination.

So, what's the best order?

Raw meat must be placed at the fridge's absolute bottom shelf. This is because meat packets are likely to spill away, creating a nightmare of contamination if placed on top shelf. (Still better, put meat in a bag or on a plate to catch any leaks.) Also, perishable products should be kept in the refrigerator's bottom drawers to remove them from any possible contamination with other contents in your refrigerator. And keep clean on those veggie drawers!

Pros and Cons:

Pros:

- The 'sirt foods' are expected to activate your body's sirtuin, which is a form of protein that helps to protect your cells from dying and developing diseases and controls your metabolism.
- It is based on an average sample of 40 gym-goers who each lost 7 lbs. in a week without losing muscle mass
- You may regularly have small doses of dark chocolate and wine without feeling guilty!
- It includes generally safe, nutritious foods such as buckwheat, blueberries, walnuts and green tea
- It is basically designed to keep you safe for life and to delay the aging process

Cons:

- There is a calorie limit for the first week that would no doubt cause most people to lose weight, regardless of what food they eat. This means that the participants may be losing weight due to the calorie restriction itself. For the first three days you only eat 1,000 calories a day, and then the next four days are 1,500 calories per day
- Restricting your calorie intake drastically can be dangerous if your body isn't used to it and you can feel lethargic
- There is not enough evidence that its promises,

especially the acceleration of your metabolism, are being followed through. A 40-person study is not large enough to say it will certainly work as a sustainable way to lose weight
- Only foods such as' sirt juices, rocket, soy, green tea and walnuts can be on the sirt food list.

As a consequence of the above, less focus is put on incorporating a variety of foods into your diet so you can look and feel fantastic. Eating a rainbow of fruit and veg every day, for example, means you get a range of vitamins and minerals in your meal.

Chapter 3
Best Sirtfoods

Food Names

Now that you know enough about Sirtfoods, why they're so good and what it takes to build a successful diet that will produce lifelong results, it's time to get started. So, now is the best time to get started with each of the top twenty Sirtfoods which will shortly become the basics of your daily diet.

Arugula

Clearly, Arugula (also known as rocket, rucola, rugula, and roquette) has a vivid background of American food culture. A musky green salad leaf with a prominent peppery flavor, it soon advanced from humble beginnings as the foundation of many Mediterranean farm dishes to becoming an emblem of food snobbery in many countries, thus contributing to the popularization of the word arugulance!

However, long before it became a salad leaf used in a battle of dominance, arugula became valued for its healing qualities by the ancient Greeks and Romans. Frequently used as a diuretic and nutritional aid, it earned its true renown from its notoriety for possessing strong aphrodisiac powers, so much so that arugula production was prohibited in Middle Ages monasteries, and it is also famous that the rocket fascinates the sexual appetite of drowsy men.

However, what really excites us about arugula is the booming quantities of the sirtuin-activating kaempferol and quercetin nutrients. A mixture of kaempferol and quercetin is being studied as a topical product in addition to existing sirtuin-activating effects, as together they moisten and promote collagen production in the skin. With those credentials, it's time to lose that elitist tag and consider this the leaf of preference for salad basics, where it beautifully combines with an extra virgin olive oil coating, merging to create a strong dual act of Sirtfood.

Buckwheat

Buckwheat was one of Japan's first domesticated grains, and the story tells that when Buddhist monks took long journeys into the hills, they 'd only bring a clay pot and a buckwheat bag for warmth. Buckwheat is so good that this was all they wanted, and it fed them up for weeks. Initially, because it is one of a sirtuin activator's best-known sources, called rutin, but also, because it has advantages as a cover crop, continuing to improve soil fertility and preventing growth of weeds, making it a fabulous crop for environmentally sound and sustainable agriculture.

The purpose buckwheat is head and shoulders above most other more growing grains is presumably because it's not a grain at all — it's basically a rhubarb-related fruit crop. Holding one of the largest protein contents of any plant, as well as being a Sirtfood superpower, makes it an unparalleled substitute to more widely used grains. Besides, it's as flexible as any grain goes, and by nature gluten-free. It's a perfect alternative for anyone intolerant to gluten.

Capers

In a sense, you 're not so acquainted with capers that we're discussing. Those salty, deep green, pellet-like things on top of a pizza that you may only have had opportunity to see. But certainly, they are one of the most undervalued and neglected foods out there. Excitingly, they are probably the caper bush's flower buds, which emerge extensively in the Mediterranean until being collected and stored by hand. Research now shows that capers possess essential antimicrobial, antidiabetic, anti-inflammatory, immunomodulatory, and antimicrobial activities, and have a long tradition of being used as a drug in the Mediterranean and North Africa. It's hardly shocking when we find that they are filled with components that trigger sirtuin.

We think it is about time these tiny morsels had their share of fame, too much overlooked by the other big hitters of the Mediterranean diet. Flavor-wise, it's a case of huge things coming in little bags, because they're confident they're kicking. Even if you don't know how to use them, don't get intimidated. For these diminutive nutritional superstars, when provided with the proper ingredients offer a wonderfully unique and inimitable sour / salty taste to finish off a dish in fashion, we will shortly have you excited and drop head over heels.

Celery

For centuries, Celery was around and admired — with leaves found festooning the ashes of the Egyptian pharaoh Tutankhamun who expired around 1323 BCE. Earlier varieties were very salty, and celery was commonly considered a therapeutic plant particularly for washing and detoxification to prevent disease. It is particularly important considering that liver, kidney, and gut wellbeing are among the other potential effects that research is now showing. In the seventeenth century, it was bred in captivity as a potato, and genetic engineering reduced its powerful bitter taste in favor of sweeter types, thereby securing its position as a popular salad vegetable.

It is important to keep in mind when it applies to celery, that there are two types: blanched / yellow and Pascal / green. Blanching is a methodology targeted at reducing the typical bitter taste of the celery, which has been considered to be too powerful. This entails filtering the celery before harvesting from sunshine, contributing to a paler color and a milder flavor. What a tragedy that is, for blanching dumbs down the sirtuin-activating characteristics of celery as well as dumbing down the flavor. Fortunately, the times are changing, and people are claiming actual and unique flavor and backing down to the greener wide range. Green celery is the sort that we suggest you use both in the green juices and foods, with the heart and leaves being one of the healthiest pieces.

Chilies

The chili has been an important part of gastronomic culture worldwide for hundreds of years. Towards one level it's disconcerting that we'd be so fascinated with it. Its pungent heat, caused by a material called capsaicin in chilies, is meant to inflict pain as a plant defensive measure, and dissuades predators from feeding on it, and we appreciate that. The food, and our infatuation with it, is now almost magical.

Amazingly one analysis revealed that consuming chilies together as well improves human cooperation. And from the point of view of health, we realize their alluring heat is fantastic to activate our sirtuins and enhance our metabolic processes. The culinary applications of the chili are also limitless, making it very easy to offer a strong Sirtfood raise to any meal.

While we admire not everybody is a huge admirer of hot or spicy meals, we keep hoping we can help persuade you to simply add small quantities of chilies, following recent studies suggesting that those eating spicy foods three or more times a week have a fourteen percent lower mortality rate especially in comparison to those eating them less than once a week.

The spicy the chili, the higher the Sirtfood credibility, but be careful and stay with what suits your specific needs. Serrano peppers are a perfect start-they are acceptable for many of individuals while packing heat; and for more experienced heat seekers, we suggest looking for Thai chilies for full sirtuin-activating advantages. These can be harder to locate in supermarkets but are mostly available in specialized markets in Asia. Search for deep-colored peppers, excluding any with a droopy and fuzzy feel.

Cocoa

It's no great surprise that chocolate was regarded a holy meal for ancient cultures like the Aztecs and Mayans, and was typically reserved for the elite and soldiers, served at banquets to achieve allegiance and service. Even so, there was such huge respect for the cocoa bean that this was even used as a means of exchange. It was normally served as a frothy beverage back then. Yet what might be a tastier way to get our nutritional allowance of cacao than by chocolate?

Unfortunately, there's no count here for the condensed, aged, and chemically flavored milk chocolate we usually munch. We 're talking regarding chocolate containing 85 percent solids of cocoa to gain the Sirtfood tag. But even then, apart from the amount of cocoa, not all chocolate is made equivalent. To minimize its acidity and give it a darker shade, chocolate is often processed with an alkalizing agent (known as the Dutch process). Regrettably, this phase reduces the sirtuin-activating flavanols significantly, thus severely undermining the health-promoting efficiency. Luckily, although unlike in several other nations, food labeling laws in some countries allow alkalized cocoa to be reported as such and labelled "alkali produced." They advocate preventing such items, even though they advertise a greater proportion of cocoa, and preferring rather for those that have not experienced Dutch processing to enjoy the positive effects of cocoa.

Coffee

What's all that about Sirtfood Coffee? We 're listening to you. We will tell you that there is no mistake. Gone are the days when a pang of shame had to balance our pleasure of coffee. Indeed, it is a true treasure trove of wonderful nutrients that activate sirtuin. But with more than half of developed countries, people are consuming coffee every day. Coffee boasts the commendation of becoming world number one source of polyphenols. The biggest irony is that the only thing we were admonished by so many fitness "experts" for doing was in essence the best thing we were doing about our wellbeing each day.

This is why coffee lovers have very little diabetes, and reduced costs of some cancers and neurodegenerative disease. And for the supreme joke, caffeine, rather than being a poison, positively preserves our livers and makes them safer! Yet counter to the common misconception that coffee dehydrates the body, it is now well known not to be the case, with coffee (and tea) adding very well to daily coffee drinkers' liquid intake. And, while we understand that coffee is not for everybody and some individuals might be very resilient to the negative effects of caffeine, it's good days for those who love a cup of tea or coffee.

Extra Virgin Olive Oil

Olive oil is by far the most renowned of Mediterranean dietary patterns. The olive tree is one of the oldest recorded-known domesticated trees, also known as the "immortal tree." Even though people began squeezing olives in stone mortar shells to collect them, its oil has been highly regarded, almost 7,000 years earlier. Hippocrates quoted it as a cure-all; now, a few millennia later, scientific knowledge categorically asserts its marvelous medical benefits. There is also a plethora of clinical evidence demonstrating that daily olive oil intake is strongly cardioprotective, as well as playing an active role in decreasing the incidence of significant modern-day diseases such as diabetes, other tumors, and osteoporosis, and linked to improved lifespan.

Once it comes to olive oil, the trick is to buy additional virgin to receive the benefits of Sirtfood in full. Virgin olive oil is only harvested from the fruits by mechanical action in parameters that do not contribute to the degradation of the oil, so the consistency and the polyphenol amount can be ensured. "Extra virgin" alludes to the first pressing of the fruit ("virgin" is the second pressing); it has the best taste, effectiveness, and credentials of Sirtfood, and is therefore the one that we highly suggest for using.

Garlic

Garlic has been regarded one of Nature's miracle food products for hundreds of years, with soothing and rejuvenating properties. Egyptians fed pyramid crews with garlic to increase their immune response, discourage various diseases, and enhance their effectiveness through their potential to suppress tiredness. Garlic is a potent natural antibiotic and antifungal that is sometimes used to help cure ulcers in the stomach. By accelerating the withdrawal of metabolic waste products, it can enhance the lymphatic system to "detox". So, despite being tested for weight reduction, it also delivers a powerful heart safety punch, decreasing cholesterol by around ten percent so reducing blood pressure by five to seven percent, as well as decreasing stickiness of blood and blood sugar. So, if you are concerned about the taste of garlic being off-putting, remain aware. When women were asked to determine a range of men's body odors, it was found that all men who ate four or more garlic cloves a day had a much more appealing and friendly smell. Experts suggest this is because it is regarded to be a stronger signal for wellbeing.

Eating garlic has a method to get greatest benefit. In garlic, the Sirtfood nutrients are enhanced by another main nutrient in it called allicin, that gives off the distinctive fragrance of garlic. But after physical "harm" to the bulb allicin only develops in garlic. So, when subject to temperature (cooking) or poor pH (stomach acid), its composition is halted. So, when preparing garlic, chop, thin, or crush, and then allow the mixture for about ten minutes prior to actually cooking or eating the allicin.

Green Tea (Especially Matcha)

Many would be experienced with green tea, the toast of the Orient and ever more famous in the West. Like the public consciousness of its medical benefits, green tea consumption is linked to less cancer, heart disease, kidney disease and osteoporosis. The reason that green tea is so healthy for us is largely due to its valuable content of a group of effective plant compounds called catechins, the center of attention is being a special form of sirtuin-activating catechin identified as epigallocatechin gallate (EGCG).

What's the debate about matcha, though? We like to believe of matcha on the steroids as ordinary green tea. In comparison to traditional green tea, which is processed as an infusion, it is a unique powdered green tea which is formulated by dissolving completely in water. The upshot of eating matcha is that it comprises significantly higher levels of the sirtuin-activating component EGCG than other green tea kinds. It is also defined matcha as the "absolute mentally and physically cure [which] has the potential to make one 's life completely full" if you are seeking for more encouragement.

Kale

We are cynics at heart, and we are still suspicious of what causes the new craze for health food ads. Is it science, or are the interests involved? In recent times few foods have boomed as significantly as kale on the wellbeing scene. Explained as the "lean, green brassica queen" (making a reference to its cruciferous vegetable family), this has become the chic vegetable for which all health-lovers and food bloggers are gearing up. Every October there is also a National Day of the Kale. But you don't have to wait until then to express your kale joy: there are already T-shirts, featuring trendy slogans like "Driven by Kale" and "road to Kale." This is enough for us to get the warning bells.

We've done extensive research, filled with concerns, and we have to acknowledge that our result is that kale really deserves her pleasures (even though we still don't suggest the T-shirts!). The explanation we 're pro-kale is that it contains bumper numbers of the quercetin and kaempferol sirtuin-activating compounds, rendering it a have to-include in the Sirtfood Diet and the source of our green Sirtfood drink. What's so exciting about kale is that kale is accessible anywhere, produced locally, and very inexpensive, unlike most of the typical expensive, hard-to-source, and hugely overpriced so-called superfoods!

Medjool Dates

It that come as a shock to include Medjool dates in a collection of foods that encourage weight loss and encourage health—especially when we informed you that Medjool dates comprise a whopping 66 percent sugar. Sugar doesn't have any sirtuin-activating qualities at all; rather, it has excellently-established links to obesity, heart disease, and diabetes — just the reverse of what we're looking to accomplish. But processed foods sugar is very distinct from sugar taken in a naturally supplied vehicle aligned with sirtuin-activating polyphenols: the date of the Medjool.

Medjool dates, consumed in moderation, do not really have any real significant blood-sugar-raising impacts, in absolute comparison with regular sugar. Then, consuming them is related to less diabetes and cardiac disorders. They have been a staple food worldwide for decades, and there has been an increase in medical interest in dates in recent times, which saw them rising as a possible remedy for a variety of diseases. It is where the Sirtfood Diet 's beauty and strength lie. It refutes the dogma and helps you to engage in nice stuff in moderation despite feeling uncomfortable.

Parsley

Parsley is sort of a cooking conundrum. It so often appears in dishes, so it's the only green guy too often. At good we serve a pair of chopped sprigs and tossed as an afterthought on a plate, at worst a single sprig for festive reasons only. This way, there on the plate it is always languishing even after we have stopped eating. This foodie styling stems from its conventional use in ancient Rome as a side dish for eating after foods in order to refresh inhale, rather than being part of the meal itself. And what an embarrass, because parsley is an amazing food that packs a vibrant, delicious flavor full of character.

Besides that, what makes parsley really special is that it is an essential source of sirtuin-activating nutrient apigenin, a tremendous blessing because it is found only in large quantities in other foods. Apigenin glues wondrously to the benzodiazepine receptors in our brains, enabling us to calm down and make us rest. Rack it all up and it's time we enjoyed parsley not as an omnipresent dietary confetto but as a result of our own choice to achieve the wonderful medical advantages it can offer.

Red Endive

Endive is a fairly new kid on the block in so far as vegetables go. History has it that a Belgian farmer found endive in 1830, by mistake. The farmer processed chicory roots in his storeroom, and then used them as a sort of coffee substitute, only to overlook about them. Upon his arrival he noticed that white leaves had started growing, which he considered to be soft, crunchy, and very tasty upon eating that. Endive has been grown throughout the world, such as the USA, and earns its Sirtfood tag thanks to its remarkable sirtuin enhancer luteolin material. And besides the proven sirtuin-activating effects, luteolin intake has become an effective option to therapy to improve socialization in autistic children.

It has a pleasing appearance and a sweet taste for those fresh to endive, followed by a gentle and friendly bitterness. If you're ever entangled on how to boost endive in your meal, you can't lose by having to add her foliage to a salad where its welcome, tart flavor adds a great bite to an extra virgin olive oil coating based on zesty. Red is great, much like onion, but the yellow kind can also be called a Sirtfood. So, whereas the red range may sometimes be more challenging to find, you can absolutely guarantee that yellow is an entirely acceptable substitute.

Red Onions

Since the time of our prehistoric ancestors, onions have been a super food, being one of the first vegetables to be grown, around 5,000 years ago. For such a lengthy tradition of use, and such strong health-giving qualities, many societies that came before us have honored onions. They were held particularly by the Egyptians as subjects of devotion, considering their circle-within-a-circle form as indicative of eternal afterlife. And the Greeks assumed that onions made athletes stronger. Athletes will eat their way through large quantities of onions before the games, even drinking the juice! It's an amazing testament to how important traditional dietary knowledge can be when we remember that onions deserve their 20 largest Sirtfood status because they're chock-full of the sirtuin-activating compounds quercetin — the very component that the sports science industry has recently started aggressively studying and promoting to boost athletic performance.

And why the red ones? Obviously because they have the higher concentration of quercetin, but the regular yellow ones do not fall far behind and are also a great selection.

Red Wine

Any majority of the top twenty Sirtfoods will not be

effective without the addition of the original Sirtfood, red wine. The French phenomenon gained notoriety in the early 1990s, with it being revealed that despite the French trying to do something wrong when it related to wellbeing (cigarettes, lack of physical activity and expensive eating habits), they had lower death rates from cardiovascular disease than countries like the United States. The justification for this was recommended by doctors was the extensive amount of red wine drunk. Danish research teams then written research in 1995 to illustrate that low-to - moderate usage of red wine decreased mortality rate, whereas roughly the same level of beverage alcohol had no impact, and comparable consumption of hard liquors continued to increase mortality rate. Obviously, in 2003, the fertile quality of red wine from a bevy of sirtuin-activating components was discovered, and the rest, as they claim, was made history.

Danish research groups then published work in 1995 to show that low to moderate use of red wine lowered mortality rates, while there was no effect on about the same level of drinking alcohol, and analogous hard liquor use tended to raise mortality rates. Evidently, in 2003, the fertile standard of red wine was identified from a bevy of sirtuin-activating ingredients, and the rest, as they say, have become history. Holding up to one 5-ounce drink a day for females and up to two 5-ounce drinks a day for males under US standards. Wines from the many region (especially pinot noir, cabernet sauvignon, and merlot) have the maximum polyphenol content among the most commonly accessible wines to guarantee greater sirtuin-activating bang for your buck.

Soy

Soy products have a long tradition as an important part of a healthy diet of many nations in Asia-Pacific such as China, Japan, and Korea. Research teams first switched on to soy after discovering that high soy-consuming countries had considerably lower incidence of many cancers, particularly breast and prostate cancers. It is believed to be due to a special class of polyphenols found in soybeans known as isoflavones, that can positively affect how estrogens function in the body that include the daidzein and formononetin sirtuin-activators. Soy oil intake has also been related to a decrease in the occurrence or intensity of a number of diseases such as heart disease, effects of menopause and bone loss.

Highly refined, nutritionally stripped soybean formulations are now a common component applied to various packaged foods. The advantages are gained either from actual soy products such as tofu, an outstanding provider of vegan protein, or in fortified form such as tempeh, natto, or our favorite, miso, a typical Japanese paste fortified with a naturally present fungus that ends in an extreme umami taste.

Strawberries

In recent times, fruit has been particularly vilified, having a poor reputation amid the rising fervor for sugar. Luckily, such a malignant image couldn't be more undeserved for berry-lovers. Although all berries are giants of protein, strawberries are winning their 20 largest Sirtfood status owing to their excess of the fisetin sirtuin activator. And now research advocate daily eating strawberries to encourage healthier longevity, keeping off Alzheimer's, obesity, diabetes, cardiovascular disease, and osteoporosis. As for their nutritional value, a mere tablespoon per 3 1/2 ounces is very small.

Amusingly, and intrinsically low in sugar itself, strawberries have created special on how the body responds to carbohydrates. What studies have discovered is that adding strawberries to carbohydrates decreases the need for insulin, effectively transforming the meal into a constant sugar releaser. Yet recent work also shows that consuming strawberries in diabetes treatment has close results to the opioid therapy.

Turmeric

Turmeric, a derivative of ginger, is the latest kid in health foods on the block. While we are just switching to it now here in the West, it has been valued for hundreds of years in Asia, for both nutritional and therapeutic applications. Amazingly, India is generating almost the entire world's turmeric stock, eating 80 % of the total of its itself. In Asia, turmeric is being used to treat skin diseases like acne, psoriasis, skin irritation and rash. Prior to actually Indian weddings, there is a celebration where the turmeric paste is implemented as a skin skincare routine to the bride and groom but also to represent the warding off misery.

One factor that prevents turmeric 's potency is that the main sirtuin-activating compound, curcumin, is badly absorbed into the body when we consume it. Research, however, reveals that we all can overcome this by preparing it in liquid, introducing fat and utilizing black pepper, all of which boost its uptake significantly. This suits well with Indian culture cuisine, where ghee and black pepper are traditionally mixed in sauces and other hot dishes, and once again proves that research just matches up with the age-old experience of conventional methods of feeding.

Walnuts

Going all the way back to 7000 BCE, walnuts are the world's oldest man-made tree product, emerging in ancient Persia, where they were the property of nobility. Fast forward to present day, and walnuts are a big success in the US. California is leading the way, with California's Central Valley famous for being the prime walnut-growing area. California walnuts also provide United States with ninety percent of market production and a whopping three-quarters of nationwide walnut production.

Walnuts pave the way as the number one nut for wellbeing. That actually makes walnuts stand out for us is how they stick out against mainstream wisdom: they are high in nutrients, but very well-established for weight reduction and the threat of biochemical diseases such as heart disease and diabetes being reduced. That is the strength of activating the sirtuin.

The recent literature revealing walnuts to be an effective anti-aging nutrient is less well known but equivalently fascinating. Evidence also refers to their advantages as a brain food with the ability to slow down brain ageing and lower the risk of debilitating brain diseases, as well as reducing the deterioration in physical activity with time.

Diet Boosting Foods

Avocado

Protein amount	Quantity of product
2 g	Each half avocado

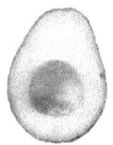

This fruit contains all 9 essential amino acids, plus cardiac omega-3 fatty acids.

Milk

Protein amount	Quantity of product
9-10 g	One cup

Milk does a healthy body, really. As well as packaging in plenty of protein, milk is also a great source of nutrients that builds bones.

Cheese

Protein amount	Quantity of product
7 g	1 ounce

Yeah, cheese can be part of a balanced diet — until you overindulge. Adhere to a serving size; combine it with an apple for an ultra-healthy appetizer.

Tempeh

Protein amount	Quantity of product
15 g	Half cup

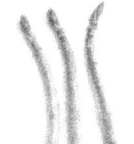

The kit kat-like texture makes the seitan a stand-in for smart meat. Salt over salads or chopped tempeh.

Asparagus

Protein amount	Quantity of product
4 g	One cup

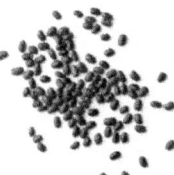

This tasty veggie is a powerhouse in nutrients. Enjoy it steamed or grilled, or scatter seeds in salads.

Black beans

Protein amount	Quantity of product
7-9 g	Half cup

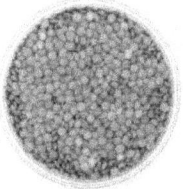

Enlist the black beans with rice or quinoa for a full protein meal.

Lentils

Protein amount	Quantity of product
9 g	½ cup

Nutritionist Marjorie Nolan Cohn, New York City owner

of MNC Nutrition, reaches out for foods high in resistant starch, a special fiber type. "The small intestine does not digest resistant starch, meaning it reaches the whole of the large intestine where it ferments," she says. " This method involves beneficial fatty acids which might obstruct the person's ability to burn carbohydrates, and instead it uses recently eaten stored body fat and fat as fuel."

Greek yogurt

Protein amount	Quantity of product
18 g	6 oz

This rich and creamy treat contains almost twice as much protein as other sources of milk; it is perfect with fruit.

Tree nuts

Protein amount	Quantity of product
4-6 g	2 tablespoons

A small pound of walnuts or almonds is great as a sweet treat, mixed in yogurt or a salad.

Edamame

Protein amount	Quantity of product
8.5 g	Half cup

An individually packaged packs almost every trace of mineral needed by your body, including iron, magnesium and zinc.

Whey protein

Protein amount	Quantity of product
24 g	1 oz

For a fast protein hit, add a scoop to the smoothies or water. Avoiding feeding stuffs? Try protein powder on soy.

Spinach

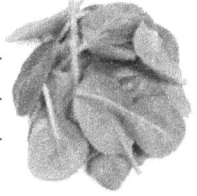

Protein amount	Quantity of product
5 g	1 cup (cooked)

Spinach boasts the highest protein content, of all the leafy greens. Try sautéing it with a little garlic.

Tofu

Protein amount	Quantity of product
12 g	3 oz

This low-calorie, flexible protein is made from soybeans and will take on any flavor, from Asian to barbecue.

Fish and shellfish

Protein amount	Quantity of product
28 g	4 oz

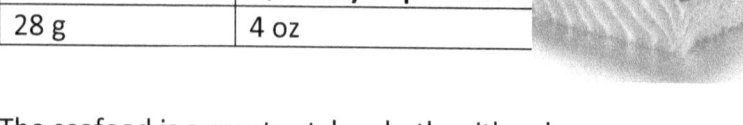

The seafood is a great catch, whether it's salmon, halibut or tuna. Target 3 to 5 servings per week.

Pseudo grains

Protein amount	Quantity of product
5-9 g	1 cup(cooked)

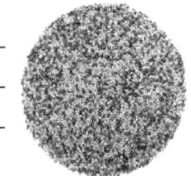

These hearty, grainy seeds (quinoa, amaranth, and buckwheat) contain more protein than cor wheat.

Chickpeas

Protein amount	Quantity of product
15 g	1 cup

Brush them as a snack, add them to a salad or throw them in the food processor for a hummus recipe.

Eggs

Protein amount	Quantity of product
12 g	2 eggs
14 g	4 white eggs

Eggs and egg whites are smart food for muscles however you prepare them. (Take a look at these healthy morning breakfasts ideas.)

Poultry and pork

Protein amount	Quantity of product
28 g	4 oz

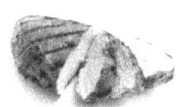

Family faves like skinless chicken and pork make every meal easy to score enough protein.

Hemp seeds

Protein amount	Quantity of product
11 g	3 tablespoons

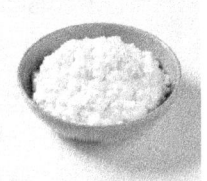

Sprinkle the hemp seeds on rice, smoothies or salads for an extra crunch.

Cottage cheese

Protein amount	Quantity of product
25 g	1 cup

For a sweet and satisfying breakfast combine cottage cheese with berries or pineapple. A word of warning: Cottage cheese can be high in sodium, so carefully read the labels.

Chapter 4:
How to Build Muscles

One surprising result from our prospective study that really puzzled us was that the respondents' muscle mass did not drop; instead, it rose by just over one pound on average. Although it was normal losing seven pounds, we have seen something interesting happening too. The losses on the measurements certainly appeared extra disheartening than this for just about two-thirds of our attendees, while still very remarkable, with a weight reduction of just over five lbs. But when experiments were conducted on body shape, we were astonished. In these attendees' muscle mass was not only maintained, it had enhanced. The total muscle growth for this category was almost two pounds, adding seven pounds to what is called a "muscular-gain-based weight loss."

This was totally shocking and in marked contrast to what usually occurs on diets with weight-loss, where individuals lose some fat but also lose muscle strength.

For any diet which reduces kcal, it's the traditional trade-off: you say good-bye muscle and also fat. It is not at all shocking when you know that cells change from growth phase to defense mode as we starve the body of nutrition and can use the protein from the muscles as food.

Sirtuins and Muscles Mass

Within the body, there is a group of genes that function as defenders of our muscles and when undergoing stress avoid its collapse: the sirtuins. SIRT1 is a strong Muscle Degradation Antagonist. As long as SIRT1 is triggered, muscle deterioration is stopped even when we're fasting, so we start to burn fat for energy.

But SIRT1 's advantages aren't done with maintaining lean muscle. In fact, the sirtuins improve and increase our skeletal muscle strength and mass. We ought to delve into the fascinating world of stem cells to illustrate how the process works. Our muscles include a particular form of stem cell which is called a satellite cell that regulates its development and reconstruction. Much of the period, satellite cells just sit in silence, but they are powered up when the muscle gets broken or stressed. Through things like weightlifting this is how our muscle grow stronger. SIRT1 is important for triggering satellite cells, so muscles are considerably weaker without their operation since they no longer have the ability to fully grow or repair. Even then, we are giving more power to our satellite cells by rising SIRT1 activation which promotes muscle growth and repair.

Sirtfoods VS Fasting

This points to a major question: if activation of the sirtuin enhances muscle strength, why do we lose more muscle when we fast? Fasting also stimulates our sirtuin genes, and besides. And therein is one of fasting 's big disadvantages.

Not all structural muscles are made equal to each other. We have two key forms, called type-1 and type-2 surprisingly. Type-1 muscle is being used for movements of prolonged period, while the type-2 muscles are used for brief periods with more strenuous exercise. But here it gets fascinating: Fasting even tends to increase SIRT1 action in muscle fibers type-1, not type-2. So, the size of the type-1 muscle fiber is preserved and even increases exponentially if we are fasting. Unfortunately, in absolute comparison to what occurs throughout fasting in type-1 fibers, SIRT1 decreases quickly in type-2 fibers. This indicates the fat burning comes to a halt, and muscles breaks down with aim of providing heat, respectively.

And, for muscles tissues, fasting will be a double-edged knife, with our type-2 fibers getting a kick. Type-2 fibers make up the bulk of our description of muscles. But even though our type-1 fiber mass is increasing, with fasting we still see a substantial expected loss of muscles. If we were able to avoid the collapse, it would not only make us all look artistically healthy but also hopefully encourage more loss of weight. And the way to do this is to fight the drop in SIRT1 in muscle fiber type-2 that is caused by fasting.

Scientists brought this to the test in an interesting mice trial and found that throughout fasting the triggers for glycogen depletion were turned off by inducing SIRT1 activity in type-2 fibers and no muscle damage occurred.

The investigators then took a step forward and checked the impact on the musculature of elevated SIRT1 activation when the mice were feed rather than felt hungry and found that it caused very massive development of the muscles. In a week, muscle cells with elevated levels of SIRT1 activation displayed an impressive weight gain of twenty percent.

These research results are very comparable to the end result of our Sirtfood Diet trial, though in impact, our study has been relatively mild. By enhancing SIRT1 activity and consuming a diet rich in sirtfoods, most respondents had no muscle damage — and for others, it was just a mild strong, muscle mass that increased substantially.

Keeping Muscles Young

And this is not just the thickness of the body. SIRT1's extensive impact on the body apply to the way it operates too. When the muscle ages it loses its capacity to trigger SIRT1. This renders it less sensitive to workout effects and more vulnerable to reactive oxygen species and inflammatory destruction, resulting in what is known as oxidative stress. Progressively muscles turn down, weaker, and easier tiredness. But if we can boost SIRT1 activation, we can prevent the downward trend associated with ageing.

Nevertheless, through triggering SIRT1 to avoid the loss of muscle mass and activity we usually see with aging process, we see contains several different medical benefits, like stopping bone loss and avoiding increased chronic systemic inflammation (known as inflammation), as well as increases in agility and general quality of life. So, interestingly, the new study shows that the higher the polyphenol level (and hence sirtuin-activating nutrients) in older individual's diets, the growing the security they benefit against deteriorating physical activity with aging.

Don't be misled into believing that such incentives extend only to the aged; far from that. Around the age of twenty-five, the symptoms of ageing will begin, and the muscles gradually destroys, with ten percent of the muscles losing by the age of forty (although average weight continues to increase) and a loss of forty percent by age 70. Yet there is considerable evidence that the activation of our sirtuin genes will inhibit and undo all of this.

Loss of muscle, development, and feature: sirtuin activity plays a crucial role in all of this. Pile it up, and it's no surprise that sirtuins were presented as point increase of muscle building in a recent analysis in the prestigious medical journal Nature, with rising sirtuin stimulation cited as one of the enabling faster avenues for battling loss of muscle mass, thus going to increase the standard of living, as well as lessening sickness and mortality.

Considered in the light of the strong impact our sirtuin genetics can have on the muscle, our prototype trial's surprise findings no longer appeared so surprising. We began to realize that spurring weight loss while trying to feed our muscle groups was feasible, all through a balanced diet in Sirtfood.

But this is only the beginning. We'll discuss Sirtfoods' advantages going so much more, to all facets of health and quality of life.

SUMMARY

- Even after weight loss we find that individual either retained or even added muscle during the Sirtfood Diet. This is because sirtuins are chief muscle controllers.
- By triggering the sirtuins, muscle collapse can be prevented, and muscle restoration promoted.
- SIRT1 activation can also assist to avoid the significant deterioration of muscle that we see

with ageing.
- Triggering your sirtuin genetics will not only make you appear leaner but will also assist you to remain healthy and productive well as you mature.

Chapter 5
Build a Diet That Works

Tips to build the sirtfood diet that better fits for you

We have done something very unique with the Sirtfood Diet. We took the most powerful Sirtfoods on the biosphere and knitted them into a brand-new healthy diet, the likes of which were not seen before. We picked the "best and brightest" from the healthful diets we have ever identified and built a world-beating recipe from them.

The great thing is you don't immediately have to follow an Okinawan 's typical diet or eat like an Italian mamma. This on the Sirtfood Diet is not only utterly unfeasible, but also needless. Yes, one thing you may be taken by from the Sirtfoods list is their similarity. While you do not consume any of the items on the list at the moment, you are very much probably eating others. And why don't you just lose weight already?

The issue is addressed when we analyze the

various elements that the most chopping-edge nutrition science displays are required to build a workable diet. It is about eating proper amount of Sirtfoods, range and shape. It's about adding ample protein portions to the Sirtfood bowls, and then enjoying your foods at the right time of day. And it's about the freedom to eat the genuinely savory foods you love in the quantities you admire.

Hitting Your Quota

Most people just don't eat nearly sufficient Sirtfoods right now to evoke a strong fat-burning and fitness-boosting influence. When study looked at the utilization in the US diet of five main sirtuin-activating components (quercetin, luteolin, myricetin, kaempferol, and apigenin), human dietary intakes were found to be miserably thirteen milligrams a day. Conversely, the Japanese daily consumption was 5 times greater. Contrasting that with our Sirtfood Diet experiment, where every day persons ate hundreds of milligrams of sirtuin-activating foods.

All we are speaking about is a true diet transformation in which we raise by as much as 50 times our daily consumption of sirtuin-activating components. Although that might seem overwhelming or unrealistic, it isn't necessarily. By taking all our highest level Sirtfoods and trying to put them together in a manner that is fully consistent with your stressful schedule, you can indeed efficiently and cheaply reach the level of consumption needed to gain all of the advantages.

The Power of Synergy

We think it is important to eat a vast array of these wonder nutrients as organic whole foods, where they coexist along with the dozens of other natural biologically active substances that work synergistically to increase our wellbeing. We think working with natural world is best, instead of against. This is for this purpose that single nutrient supplementation does not display permanent effect time and time again, but the same component is represented in the form of an entire diet.

Take, for example, the basic component resveratrol which activates sirtuin. This is partially consumed in supplementary form; but its bioavailability (how much more the individual can use) is at least 6 times higher in its normal food material of red wine. Refer to this the reality that red wine produces not only one but a complete variety of sirtuin-activating polyphenols that work with each other to offer positive effects, like myricetin, piceatannol, quercetin and epicatechin. Perhaps we could direct our focus from the turmeric to curcumin. Curcumin is very well-established as the main sirtuin-activating ingredient in turmeric, but work reveals that this whole turmeric has stronger PPAR-ÿ action to combat fat burning and is much more capable of suppressing cancer and decreasing blood glucose levels than isolated curcumin. It's not hard to understand that trying to isolate a single nutrient in its full food process is still nowhere near as successful as eating it.

Yet when we begin combining multiple Sirtfoods, what really makes a nutritional plan special is. For example, by trying to introduce it in quercetin-rich Sirtfoods we enhance the impacts of resveratrol-containing foods a lot further. Not even just that even in their conduct they complement one another. All of those are fat blockers, but how either of them actually achieves that is complicated. Resveratrol is very effective in promoting deterioration of mature fat cells, while quercetin is active in preventing new fat tissue from developing. In addition, they ingest food on both ends, leading to a high losing weight impact than consuming just large amounts of a single ingredient.

So, this is a method which we see again and again. Foods that are high in sirtuin enhancer apigenin boost the quercetin uptake from diet and increase its function. Quercetin in effect has been shown to be synergistic with epigallocatechin gallate (EGCG) activity. And EGCG 's work with curcumin has been seen to be complementary. And so, it begins. Not only are individual whole products more effective than single ingredients, but we reach into yet another tapestry of beneficial effects that natural world has blended — so deep, so pure, it's difficult to attempt to beat it.

Juicing and Food: Get the Best of Both Worlds

Sirtfood Diet is portion of both juices and whole food products. There we are speaking about juices made directly from a juicer — blenders and milkshake makers (including the NutriBullet) do not work. For others that may sound counterintuitive, based on the fact that the fiber is lost while it is juiced. Yet this is just what we need from leafy green vegetables.

Feed fiber includes what is termed non-extractable polyphenols (or NEPPs). Which are polyphenols, called sirtuin additives, which are bound to the fibrous portion of the food and only emitted by our helpful intestinal bacteria when decomposed. We don't even get the NEPPs by erasing the fiber and end up losing out on their righteousness. Crucially, though, the NEPP composition varies significantly based on the size of the plant. The NEPP material of diet rich in fruits, cereals, and grains is meaningful and should be ingested whole (NEPPs provide over fifty percent of polyphenols in strawberries!). However, for leafy green vegetables, the essential compounds in the Sirtfood juice, they are much lesser even after having a bigger fiber content.

So, we get full value for our buck whenever it applies to leafy green vegetables by juicing them and eliminating the low-nutrient material, so we can use even increasing quantities and obtain an amazingly concentrated dose of sirtuin-activating polyphenols.

There is yet another benefit of cutting the fibers, too. Green leafy vegetables contain a form of fiber called non - soluble fiber which has a gastrointestinal scrubbing action. However, when we consume so much of it, it will frustrate and hurt our digestive lining quite as if we over-scrub stuff. That ensures that for so many people, green leafy vegetables-packed smoothies can overwhelm fibred, possibly aggravating or even inducing IBS (irritable bowel syndrome) and hampering our nutrient uptake.

When it tends to come to digesting their goodness, having a few of your Sirtfoods in juice form can even have significant benefits. For instance, matcha green tea has been one of the additives we include that in the green juice. When we eat the EGCG sirtuin activator present in high amounts of green tea in the form of drinks lacking milk, its ingestion is higher than sixty-five percent. We also found it important to remember that transitioning towards smoothies to green juices carried about significant rises in their quantities of other vital nutrients, including such magnesium and folic acid, as we ran lab tests on our own customers.

The core issue of it all is that to get those sirtuin genetic factors ringing for massive weight loss and wellbeing, we have to establish an eating plan that incorporates for greatest advantage both juices and whole meals.

The Power of Protein

These are plants that bring the Sirt into the nutrition of Sirtfood, yet to get optimum value,

Sirtfood foods will also have a high protein content. Has shown that a major component of the dietary specific protein leucine has extra advantages in enhancing SIRT1 to enhance fat loss and boost blood sugar regulation.

But leucine now has another role, and that's where it genuinely glows through its balanced interaction with Sirtfoods. Leucine effectively induces anabolism (building things) in our cells, especially in the muscle, which requires a great deal of energy and ensures that our energy producers (called mitochondria) have to work extra hours. It induces the need for such a Sirtfoods operation within our cells. As you may actually remember, one of the impacts of Sirtfoods is to increase the growth of more mitochondria, to increase their efficiency, and to make them blow fat as fuel. Our bodies therefore need these to fulfill this extra demand for energy. The truth of the matter is that we see a synergistic impact when mixing Sirtfoods with dietary protein that enhances sirtuin activation and eventually allows you to lose fat to support muscle development and better safety. Of this reason the meals in the guide are built to have a reasonable protein portion.

Oily fish are an incredibly strong protein

alternative to supplement Sirtfoods' action since they are high in omega-3 fatty acids alongside their nutritional value. There is no way that you may have read a lot about the health effects of oily fish and especially omega-3 fish oils. And now new evidence shows that the advantages of omega-3 fats may come from improving the functioning of our sirtuin genomes.

In recent times, questions have been presented about the harmful impact of protein-rich diets on wellbeing, without any Sirtfoods to help counter the protein, we can come to recognize why. Leucine may be a knife with two-edges. We need Sirtfoods, as we have shown, to support our cells fulfill the metabolic requirements that leucine imposes upon them. Without them, though, our mitochondria may become unstable, so elevated rates of leucine will potentially encourage obesity so insulin tolerance, rather than boost safety. Sirtfoods support not only keep the symptoms of leucine in control but also work effectively in our favor. Assume of leucine as tapping your foot on the losing weight and wellbeing accelerator, with Sirtfoods the device that guarantees that the cell fulfills the increased competition. The engine blew up, without any of the Sirtfoods.

Returning to worries about the safety consequences of protein-rich diets, the missing part of the equation is Sirtfoods. Usually, the most nations diet is protein-rich but lacks Sirtfoods to help counter it. That makes it imperative for Sirtfoods for becoming an essential component of how those nations feed.

Eat Early

Our ideology is superior when it comes to having a meal, preferably completing eating each day by 7 p.m. That is on two grounds. Firstly, to enjoy the Sirtfoods natural satiating power. Eating food that will leave you feeling full, happy, and energetic as you go about your day is even more effective than enduring the whole day feeling hungry enough to feed and stay full while having sleep throughout the night.

Yet there's a second good explanation to maintain dietary behaviors in line with your own body clock. We all have an internal body clock, called our circadian clock, which controls all of our normal functioning of the body as per daytime. It affects, inter alia, how the body processes the food we eat. Our clocks work in synchronization, above all trying to follow the signs of the sun's light-dark cycle. We're programmed as a diurnal organism to be effective in the daylight rather than at nighttime. Our body clock therefore gets us to permit access most effectively during the day, whenever it's light and we're intended to be active, and far less so when it's dark, where we're prepared for proper sleep conversely.

The question is that all of us have "work clocks" and "social clocks," which are not aligned with the sun's slowing down. Even after dusk is the last option any of us get to sleep. To some extent, we can equip our circadian rhythm to synchronize with rotating shifts, like "evening chronotypes" that favor or need to be effective, eat properly and sleep later in the day. Person who lives distorted from the light-dark exterior cycle however comes with a price. Research shows that people in the evening chronotype have increases the susceptibility to gain of body fat, muscle atrophy and metabolic disorders, as well as often having sleep deprivation. That's precisely what we see between other night shift workers, who probably have higher prevalence of obesity and metabolic disorders, at least partly due to the impacts of their delayed dietary behaviors.

The fact of the matter is that where necessary, you 're best off eating early in the day, preferably by 7 p.m. But what if it is actually not possible? The great news is that sirtuins play a key part in synchronizing the circadian rhythm. Work has actually shown that the polyphenols in Sirtfoods are able to modulate our body rhythms and change circadian rhythm favorably. Which implies the addition of Sirtfoods with your meal will mitigate the adverse consequences if you actually cannot quit consuming food later on. Evidently, one of the recurring reviews we hear from Sirtfood Diet supporters is how often their sleep pattern has continued to improve, trying to suggest significant impacts on their body clock harmonization.

Go Big on Taste

A basic problem with current eating habits is that it usually makes the eating experience uncomfortable. It flushes every little drop of food enjoyment and leaves us feeling bitter. But for us, it's important that in maintaining a healthier weight you retain the pleasure of food. That's why we were happy when we noticed that Sirtfoods and the food products that improve their action like protein and omega-3 sources of food are prepared to satisfy our flavor willingness. It's the overall win-win: The Sirtfood diet is boosting our wellbeing and wonderful tastes.

Let's go back one stage to see how all this works. Our sense of taste evaluates how delicious we probably have found our food, and how comfortable we are to consume it. This is accomplished by 7 main receptors to the taste. Human beings have developed over hundreds of generations to pursue out the flavors that enhance these receptors to reach optimal nutrition out of our diet. The more those flavor receptors are activated by a food, the more pleasure we get from a dinner. So, we have the perfect list for satisfied sense of taste in the Sirtfood Diet, as it delivers full relaxation to all taste receptors. To evaluate these tastes and the foods you'll have to eat on the diet menu that please them: the 7 major sensations of taste are sweet (strawberries, dates); sour (strawberries); bitter (cocoa, kale, extra virgin olive oil, endive green tea); stingy (chilies, garlic, extra virgin olive oil); salty (celery, fish); astringent (green tea, red wine); and umami (soy, fish, meat).

How much we have found is that the higher a food's sirtuin-activating entities, the stronger it enhances those flavor centers, and the more satisfaction we get from the food we consume. Crucially, it also ensures our hunger is met sooner, and our urge to consume more is that appropriately. That is a primary explanation why those eating a Sirtfood-rich diet are quicker happily fuller.

Organic cocoa, for instance, has a hitting, enticing sour aftertaste, but erase the sirtuin-activating flavanols with aggressive industrial food products, and we're decided to leave with density-produced, uninteresting, and charmless cocoa which is used to make extremely sweetened chocolate pastries. The beneficial effects have disappeared by this point.

The same is true of olive oil. Absorbed in its moderately refined form — extra virgin — it has a strong and unique taste which can be sensed at the back of the tongue with a hard blow. Yet refined and processed olive oil starts to lose all theme, is moderate and tasteless and does not carry a kick like this. Likewise, hot chilies hold much more sirtuin-activating credibility than the relatively mild kinds, and wild strawberries are much more tasteful than domesticated ones due to a stronger sirtuin-activating nutritional value.

Perhaps not that, we often seek that specific Sirtfoods can stimulate various receptors of flavor: green tea is both unpleasant and astringent, and strawberries combine sweet and savory flavors.

Originally, some palates won't get used to some of these flavours — much more of our industrial diets is devoid both of nutrients and genuine taste — but you'll be surprised at how fast you gain affection for them. And besides, humans are wired to look for a healthy diet in Sirtfoods, along with healthy protein and omega-3 fatty acids, to gratify our appetite's base instincts and, in turn, our wellbeing. This process of evolution has been going on for millennia without us understanding the cause, yet it has guaranteed that we get the greatest return from eating such foods.

Embrace Eating

Let's try an experiment. We always want you to do one very easy thing for us: don't dream about a polar bear.

What do you think? Of course, a polar bear. Why? For what? Even though we told you they didn't. Don't tell us you're still going to think!

It was the innovating survey performed in 1987 by psychology professor Daniel Wegner, which displayed that compelled repression of thoughts leads to a contradictory and ineffective intensification in how often we personally believe about what we are attempting to hide. So rather than obstructing it from our thought processes, the activity generates a concern for the inhibited thought.

Yet as you've already noticed, this trend doesn't even refer to polar bears. The very same thing occurs when we are making antagonists and limiting weight losing diet products. Research shows that in fact we believe more often about them, going to increase the desire. It's chewing again, before we consume it! And with the diet disrupted and the escalating anxiety of the "forbidden" foods humans' endured; we're far more likely to consume now.

Now the physicists have clarified what's going on here. We also need to be fully autonomous. When we feel restricted, like going on a limited diet, this causes a bad atmosphere which makes us feel uncomfortable. We get wrapped up in this misery and we fight to get out. We take up arms by doing what we've been told we shouldn't be doing and doing it a lot more than we would have had at first. It occurs to us all, for even the most self-controlled ones. It's not a case of when but if. Researchers now agree that this is a key explanation that we can sustain foods and even see early effects but struggle to achieve long-term progress.

So, does that mean that there was no sense in trying to improve our food patterns? Are we just doomed to fail? Yes, it means, and we need to make our own optimistic, ideal decisions while making a transition to be successful. We now know that it is not though the nutritional isolation but also through dietary inclusion that we can accomplish that. Rather than concentrating your energy on the negative aspects of what you shouldn't eat, conversely look at the positive aspects of what you should eat. You stop the social reaction by doing so. And the Sirtfood Diet's elegance is this. It's just what you placed in your meal and not what you're throwing out. This is about the reliability and not the amount of your meals. So, it's about you desiring to do anything because you feel fulfilled trying to eat great-tasting food products with the additional knowledge that every chomp provides a treasure of advantages.

Many diets represent a way to an end. They 're about keeping in there, trying to make sense of the "thin dream." However, at the end of the day, it never happens until the diet fails, so it's never maintained, even if reached. There's a special Sirtfood Diet. It's all about travelling. Phase 1, which reduces calories, is held deliberately short and quick to ensure positive effects are done before the adverse reaction happens. The emphasis then is exclusively on Sirtfoods. So, the desire to eat Sirtfoods isn't just motivated by an end product of weight loss. Now it's just as often, if not more, about appreciating and celebrating natural food for a safe and healthy lifestyle.

What's often more, once you gain Sirtfoods' useful benefits, from satisfying your desire to enhancing your quality of life, you'll find your habits and tastes variation. On the Sirtfood Diet, items that would have traditionally set off the chain of adverse responses if you had been told that you couldn't consume them would reduce their attraction and lessen their influence on you. They now become small component of the balanced diet and they have all been accomplished without a random straight bear sighting.

SUMMARY

- The Sirtfood Diet draws on the earth's most effective SIRTfoods and puts them together in such an easy and realistic way to feed.
- In order to obtain optimum performance in order to lose weight and wellbeing, Sirtfoods should be consumed in the correct amount, mixture, and formulations to gain the stimulatory activity of their sirtuin-activating chemicals.
- We even farther improve this by including most quality foods such as leucine-rich protein sources and oily fish, to start making the Sirtfood Diet 's impacts even more potent.
- Nutrition early in the day is also vital and generally keeps us in sync with our built-in circadian rhythm.
- Unlike our traditional diets, Sirtfoods satisfies all of our sweet taste, meaning that we get more pleasure from our meals and feel satisfied way quicker.
- Sirtfood diet is a participation diet – not a restriction diet, trying to make it the only form of diet that can supply long-term weight-loss achievement.

Phase 1: 7 Pounds in Seven Days

Encourage to Sirtfood Diet, Phase 1. This is the step of high energy-success, where you are going to take a big step towards accomplishing a thinner and slimmer body. Following our easy step-by - step directions and then use the tasty meals you'll find. We do have a meat-free option in comparison to our regular seven-day schedule which is ideal for vegetarians and vegans alike. Free yourself to go with whatever you chose.

What to Expect

You'll receive the amazing rewards of our scientifically validated strategy of losing seven pounds in 7 days during initiation phase. Yet note it involves adding strength, so don't just get caught up on the figures on the measurements. Nor should you become accustomed to going to weigh yourself every day. In reality, over the last few days of Phase 1 we always see the scales starting to creep due to muscle boost, while waists continue to dwindle. Therefore, we want you to focus on the scales, but not be governed by them. Find out how you feel inside the reflection, if your clothes match, or if you need to push a knot on your belt. These are all excellent examples of the deeper adjustments in your body makeup.

Be known of other variations as well, such as health, energy counts and how shining your skin looks. At the nearest clinic, you can also have tests of the general diseases and cardiovascular safety and see improvements at factors like the blood rate, blood sugar rates and blood fats such as triglycerides and cholesterol. Also, losing weight aside, incorporating Sirtfoods into your diets is a big step towards making your cells fit and healthy and more disease-resistant, putting you up for an extraordinary balanced lifespan.

How to Follow Phase 1

In order to keep Phase 1 as smooth sailing as practicable, we will lead you one day at a time through the whole seven-day cycle, along with the full rundown on the Sirtfood green smoothie and easy-to - follow, tasty meals every inch of the process.

Stage 1 of the Sirtfood Diet consists of two distinct phases:

Days 1 to 3 Are the most computationally intense, and you can consume up to thousand calories per day during this time frame, comprised of:

- 3 x Sirtfood green vegetable juices
- 1 x main diet

Days 4 to 7 You can see your caloric intake rise to a daily limit of fifteen hundred calories, composed of:

- 2 x Sirtfood green vegetable juices

- 2 x main diets

There are so few rules by which to obey the diet. Undoubtedly, for sustained progress, it's about incorporating it into the routine and around the daily life. But here are a few straight forwards yet large-impact recommendations to get the best result:

1: Get a Good Juicer: Fruit juice is an essential part of the Sirtfood nutrition, and a blender is one of the important purchases you'll make for your wellbeing. While expenditure should always be the key point, some mixers are more efficient at trying to extract the juice from leafy greens vegetables and herbs.

2: Preparation Is Key: Yet another thing is for sure from the riches of feedback we've had: those who scheduled ahead of time were the most able to succeed. Get to know the food ingredients and methods and start stocking up on what's needed. You'll be surprised at how easy the entire process is, with almost everything coordinated and prepared.

3. Save Time: If time is tight, start preparing cleverly. Food should be rendered the previous night. Liquids can be made in quantity and stored in the refrigerator for up to 3 days (or further in the refrigerator) until their sirtuin-activating nutrient uptake begin to decrease. Only shield it from glare and insert only when you're able to eat it in the matcha.

4. Eat Early: Eating fairly early in the day is nicer and preferably, food and juices should not be ingested later than 7 p.m. But the diet is essentially tailored for the routine, and late people who eat still profit greatly.

5. Space Out the Juices: In order to increase the uptake of green juices, they must be ingested at least 1 hour before or 2 hours after a diet and distributed throughout the day, instead of being too close next to each other

6. Eat until Satisfied: Sirtfoods may have serious impacts on hunger, and maybe some people will be exhausted until their diets are over. Pay attention to your body and eat till fulfilled, rather than pushing down all the meals. Say, "Hara hachi bu," as the long-lived Okinawans do, which translates literally as "Eat until you are eighty percent jam - packed."

7. Enjoy the Journey: Would not get engaged on the ultimate objective; process implementation of the adventure conversely. This diet is about commemorating food in all its mystery, for its beneficial effects but also for the pleasure and satisfaction it brings. Studies suggest that we are much better likely to be successful if we keep our eyes concentrated on the road rather than the ultimate goal.

What to Drink

And also, the required daily quantities of green juices, other drinks should be easily drinking in Phase 1. Non-calorie beverages, ideally plain juice, black coffee, and herbal tea. If your standard preferences are for dark or herbal teas, do not hesitate to include all these also. Fruit juices and carbonated beverages are rendered behind. Rather, consider adding a few sliced strawberries to still or sparkling water to make your own Sirtfood-infused health cocktail if you'd like to spice things up. Retain it for a few hours in the fridge and you will have a delightfully fascinating substitute to soft drinks and juices.

One thing you need to be conscious of is that we don't advise sudden major changes to your standard coffee use. Caffeine side effects may make you feel shockingly bad for a few days; similarly, large increases may be awkward for those especially sensitive to caffeine impacts. We also suggest drinking coffee black without putting milk, as some studies have found that adding milk will minimize the absorption of important nutrients that trigger sirtuin. 1 The same was found for green tea, 2 although adding some lemon juice definitely improves the strength of its nutrients which activate sirtuin.

Realize that this is the phase of high energy-success, and while you must be soothed by the reality that this is only for a whole week, you have to be a little more conscientious. We usually involve alcohol for last week, in the shape of red wine but only as a food preservative.

The SirtFood Green Juice

The green juice is an important component of Sirtfood Diet's Phase 1 program. All the components are strong Sirtfoods, and with each juice you get a greatest advantage of natural products like apigenin, kaempferol, luteolin, quercetin, and EGCG that function together just to turn on the sirtuin genes and encourage fat burning. To this we have applied lemon as its inherent acidity has also been shown to secure, maintain and improve the ingestion of the sirtuin-activating components of the drink. We have added a bit of apple and ginger for flavor, too. Hence all of these are available. Admittedly, several people notice that they cut out the apples entirely because they become used to the flavor of the fruit.

Green Juice Preparation (SERVES 1)

1. 2 large handfuls (about 2 1/2 ounces or 75g) kale
2. a large handful (1 ounce or 30g) arugula
3. a very small handful (about 1/4 ounce or 5g) at-leaf parsley
4. 2 to 3 large celery stalks (5 1/2 ounces or 150g), including leaves
5. 1/2 medium green apple
6. 1/2- to 1-inch (1 to 2.5 cm) piece of fresh ginger
7. juice of 1/2 lemon
8. 1/2 level teaspoon matcha powder

Days 1 to 3 of Phase 1: added only to the first two juices of the day.

Days 4 to 7 of Phase 1: added to both juices

Recognize that while we balanced all the large amounts exactly as listed in our prospective study, our perspective is that bunch of indicators work exceptionally well. In reality, they are better tailoring the quantity of nutrients to the body size of an ordinary person. Larger people tend to have a larger hand and even get a substantially greater amount of Sirtfood nutrients to meet their physical appearance and relatively small people vice versa

- Mix these greens together (kale, arugula, and parsley), and sauté them. We notice that mixers really can vary in their effectiveness when juicing leafy green vegetables, even before shifting on to the other additives, you may have to rejoice the remainder. The target is to end up with about 2 pounds of liquid or near to 1/4 cup (50ml) of green vegetable juice.
- Now juice the apple, celery, and ginger juice.
- You can also slice the lemon and placed it through the blender, but we find it a lot easier to push the lemon into the liquid by hand. You ought to have approximately 1 cup (250ml) of juices in maximum by this point, maybe much more.
- It's only after you make the juice and are capable of serving that you add the matcha. In a bowl, place a small amount of water, then insert the

matcha, and mix rapidly with a fork or tablespoon. In the first two cups of the day, we only use matcha, as it based on small levels of caffeine (the same quality as a regular teacup). If drank late, it will keep you up for those not used to it.
- Add the remaining juice, once the matcha is abolished. Give it a swirl end, and the juice becomes able to drink. Easy to top up with simple tea if you want.

Phase 1: Your Seven-Day Guide

Please be aware before cooking begins.

Take the juice at various times during twenty-four hours for Days 1 to 3 (e.g., very first thing every morning, mid-morning and late-afternoon), and choose one of the regular or vegetarian meal choices and consume them at a time and place that soothe you (generally eaten for dinner or lunch).

Day 1

On Day 1, you will consume:

- 3 x Sirtfood green juices
- 1 x main meal (standard or vegan option), either:

Asian shrimp stir-fry with buckwheat noodles

+

1/2 to 3/4 ounce (15 to 20g) dark chocolate (85 percent cocoa solids)

or

Miso and sesame glazed tofu with ginger and chili stir-fried greens (vegan)

+

1/2 to 3/4 ounce (15 to 20g) dark chocolate (85 percent cocoa solids)

Day 2

On Day 2, you will consume:

- 3 x Sirtfood green juices
- 1 x main meal (standard or vegan option), either:

Turkey escalope with sage, capers, and parsley and spiced cauliflower "couscous"

+

1/2 to 3/4 ounce (15 to 20g) dark chocolate (85 percent cocoa solids)

or

Kale and red onion dal with buckwheat (vegan)

+

1/2 to 3/4 ounce (15 to 20g) dark chocolate (85 percent cocoa solids)

Day 3

On Day 3, you will consume:

- 3 x Sirtfood green juices
- 1 x main meal (standard or vegan option), either:

Aromatic chicken breast with kale and red onions and a tomato and chili salsa

+

1 /2 to 3 /4 ounce (15 to 20g) dark chocolate (85 percent cocoa solids)

or

Harissa baked tofu with cauliflower "couscous" (vegan)

+

1 /2 to 3 /4 ounce (15 to 20g) dark chocolate (85 percent cocoa solids)

Start taking the juices at different moments of the day for days four to seven (e.g., the very first juice either in the morning or full back-morning, the second late afternoon juice); then choose your meals from either conventional or vegetarian cuisine and consume them at the right time (usually ingested for breakfast / dinner and lunch). You may also keep adding darker chocolate (eighty-five percent cocoa solids) in 1/2 to 3/4 ounces (15 to 20 g) every day, at your authority, depending on your desire to eat.

Day 4

On Day 4, you will consume:

- 2 x Sirtfood green juices
- 2 x main meals (standard or vegan option), either:

MEAL 1: Sirt muesli

MEAL 2: Pan-fried salmon fillet with caramelized endive, arugula, and celery leaf salad

or

MEAL 1: Sirt muesli (vegan)

MEAL 2: Tuscan bean stew (vegan)

Day 5

On Day 5, you will consume:

- 2 x Sirtfood green juices
- 2 x main meals (standard or vegan option), either:

MEAL 1: Strawberry buckwheat tabbouleh

MEAL 2: Miso-marinated baked cod with stir-fried greens and

sesame

or

MEAL 1: Strawberry buckwheat tabbouleh (vegan)

MEAL 2: Soba (buckwheat noodles) in a miso broth with tofu, celery, and kale (vegan)

Day 6

On Day 6, you will consume:

- 2 x Sirtfood green juices
- 2 x main meals (standard or vegan option), either:

MEAL 1: Sirt super salad

MEAL 2: Char-grilled beef with a red wine jus, onion rings, garlic kale, and herb-roasted potatoes

or

MEAL 1: Lentil Sirt super salad (vegan)

MEAL 2: Kidney bean mole with baked potato (vegan)

Day 7

On Day 7, you will consume:

- 2 x Sirtfood green juices
- 2 x main meals (standard or vegan option), either:

MEAL 1: Sirtfood omelet

MEAL 2: Baked chicken breast with walnut and parsley pesto and red onion salad

or

MEAL 1: Waldorf salad (vegan)

MEAL 2: Roasted eggplant wedges with walnut and parsley pesto and tomato salad (vegan)

Phase 2: Maintenance

Credits on finishing Sirtfood Diet Step 1! You will now have amazing progress after a weight reduction so not only look thinner and more muscular but also feel transformed and re-energized. So, what's next?

While everyone else has seen these almost always-remarkable modifications ourselves, we know what else you're going to want to see even good outcomes, not just maintain all those advantages. Sirtfoods are, after all, meant to eat for living. The issue is how you customize what you did in Phase 1 into your daily nutritional routine. This is precisely what inspired us to develop a 14-day maintenance schedule intended to help you make the shift from Phase 1 to your more daily nutritional regimen, thus helping to maintain and expand the advantages of the Sirtfood Diet deeper.

What to Expect

You will maintain the weight loss results through Step 2 and start to lose weight gradually.

Note, the one surprising point we've seen with the Sirtfood Diet is that much or all of the obese people lose is from fat, and many of those definitely contribute some strength in. Therefore, we would like to inform you again that you don't just evaluate your success by the percentages on measurement. Look into a mirror to see if you look thinner and more muscular, see how well your dress fits, and gobble up the nice comments you'll get from others.

Also remember that as the losing weight continues, so will the medical benefits. By trying to follow the 14-day maintenance program, you are indeed beginning to lay the groundwork for a long-term health for coming years.

How to Follow Phase 2

The trick to progress in this process is having your nutrition packed full of Sirtfoods. To render it as simple as possible, we have prepared a seven-day meal schedule for you to fulfill its requirements, with tasty and healthy recipes, filled with Sirtfoods every day to the rafters. All you have to do is replicate the Seven Day Schedule again to fulfill Step 2's 14 days.

On each of the fourteen days your diet will consist of:

- 3 x balanced Sirtfood-enriched meals
- 1 x Sirtfood green vegetable juice
- 1 to 2 x optional Sirtfood bite snacks

Also, when you've had to eat those, there have been no strict rules. Be agile throughout the day and follow them. Two basic thumb-rules are:

- Have your green vegetable juice either early that morning, at least thirty minutes before dawn meal, or in the middle of the dawn.

- Do your hardest to finish your dinner before 7 p.m.

PORTION SIZES

In second phase our attention is not on counting calories. For the common citizen that is not a realistic solution or even an effective one in the lengthy period. Rather we concentrate on healthy servings, quite well-balanced meals, and perhaps most importantly, loading up on Sirtfoods so that you can start to profit from their chubby-burning and health-increasing impact.

Also, we've built the food in the strategy to help satisfy them, which will made you look full and satisfied. That synchronized with Sirtfoods' natural hunger-regulating effects, means you're not going to spend the next 14 days feeling hungry, but rather generally satisfied, well-fed, and almost well-nourished.

Just like in Phase 1, listen attentively, and be directed by your desire to eat. When you prepare food as per our directions and consider that you are easily full before you have completed a meal, then quit consuming is completely acceptable!

WHAT TO DRINK

Through most of Step 2 you'll have to have one green vegetable juice daily. This is to maintain you with high Sirtfoods levels.

Much as in Phase 1, you can easily absorb certain fluids in Phase 2. Our favorite beverages comprise remaining plain beer, bottled sweet soda, coffee, and green tea. If black or white tea is your predisposition, please enjoy. The very same holds for black tea. The biggest comment is that throughout Phase 2 you can admire an occasional glass of red wine. Due to its high content of sirtuin-activating polyphenols, particularly resveratrol and piceatannol, red wine is a sirtfood which makes it by far the right alcoholic drink. But, with liquor itself causing negative impacts on our fat tissue, restraint is always safest, so we suggest restricting the drink to one glass of red wine with a food for 2 to 3 days a week during Phase 2.

RETURNING TO THREE MEALS

You ingested only one or two meals per day during Phase 1 which allowed you plenty of versatility when you eat your food. Since we are all returning to a more usual schedule and the well-tested practice of 3 meals a day, learning about breakfast is a perfect idea.

Eating nutritious breakfast tends to put us on for the day, rising our amounts of energy and focus. Eating early holds our blood glucose and fat levels in balance, in terms of our metabolism. That meal is a good thing is pointed out by a series of studies usually finding that individuals who eat breakfast often are less probable to obese.

This is because of our body's internal rhythms. Our organs are asking us to feed early in expectation of when we will be much busier and need food. Yet more than a third of us will miss breakfasts on every given day. It's a typical example of our crazy daily life and the feeling that there's just not enough room to eat properly. But as you can see, nothing could be far from the fact with the lovely meals that we have set over here for you. If it's the Sirtfood smoothie that can be drank on the go, the premade Sirt muesli, or the fast and simple Sirtfood scrambled eggs / tofu, having some additional few moments in the morning will yield rewards not only for your whole day but also for your fitness and wellbeing over the lengthy period.

Despite Sirtfoods serving to overcharge our metabolism, there's only more to learn from having a boost from them early that morning to continue your day. It is done not only by eating a Sirtfood-rich meal, but above all by consuming the green vegetable juice, which we suggest you have either first thing every morning — at least 30 minutes before meal — or lane-morning. We get a lot of stories from our own personal experience about people who first sip their green vegetable juice and don't feel thirsty for a few hours afterwards If that is the impact it has on you, waiting a few hours before eating breakfast is well. Just really don't miss this one. Conversely, with a healthy meal, you can start your day, then look for two or three hours to have the green vegetable juice. Be easy, and simply go with anything that soothes you.

SIRTFOOD BITES

You should handle it when it relates to eating or leave it. There has been too much discussion over whether eating regular, smaller meals is better for losing the weight, or only sticking to 3 healthy meals a day. The reality is that it is not really relevant.

The way we've built the servicing menu for you guarantees you 're going to eat 3 well-balanced Sirtfood-rich meals a day and you might find that you don't always need a snack. So, maybe you've been engaged with the kids in the classroom, going out or dashing about and have something to take you until the next food. But if that "little thing" will offer you a whammy of Sirtfood vitamins and minerals so wonderful to taste, then it's a good time. That's why we developed our "Sirtfood Bits." These fun little treats are a truly misery-free treat made completely from sirtfoods: almonds, walnuts, chocolate, turmeric, and extra virgin olive oil and. We suggest eating one, or a possibility of two, every other day for the days that you really need them.

"SIRTIFYING" YOUR MEALS

We found that the only consistent meals are ones of acceptance, not removal. Yet real achievement goes well beyond that — the diet needs to be consistent with life in modern times. If it's the ease of satisfying the needs of our stressful lifestyle or keeping in with our position at social events as the bon vivant, the way we feed should be trouble-free. You will admire your svelte body and beautiful smile, rather than thinking about the requirements and limitations of kooky products.

What makes Sirtfoods so fabulous is that they are really available, common, and simple to be included in your eating habits. Here, when you cross the distance between step 1 and daily feeding, you can lay the groundwork for a new, enhanced lifelong feeding strategy.

The basic feature is what we call your meal options "Sirtifying." And this is where we take popular meals, along with several classic favorite's, and we retain all the fantastic flavor with some smart swaps and easy Sirtfood additions but add a lot of stuff to that. You'll see how conveniently this is accomplished all across Phase 2.

Highlights feature our tasty smoothie Sirtfood for the ultimate on-the-go breakfast in a time-consuming universe, and the easy turn from wheat to buckwheat to bring more flavor and bite to a much-loved pasta delicious meal. In the meantime, famous, adored meals such as chili con carne and curry wouldn't even need far more transition, with Sirtfood bonanzas providing local dishes. So, who has said that junk food means bad food? When you start making it yourself, we integrate the accurate lively ingredients of a pizza and erase the culpability. There's no reason to say goodbye to pleasures either, as our soaked pancakes with fruit and dark chocolate pudding has demonstrated. It's not just a cake, it's breakfast and for you it's perfect. Easy shifts: you keep eating the food that you enjoy when maintaining a good weight and stability. And this is the Sirtfood diet movement

COOKING FOR MORE

We accept this, we also are undergoing a time of "Sirtfoods for Everyone," where meals begin, we appeal to many more mouths than one. If it's for friends or family members, the latest meals for supper as well as the Sirtfood-packed soup that we present in this process are planned with everyone in mind. But why not reap the benefits of preparing food batch food to freeze for those still preparing food for one or two to have dishes prepared for this week?

FOURTEEN-DAY MEAL PLAN

Besides our pro package, we also have a meat-free edition which is fit for consumption for vegetarians. Experiment and match with whatever you want.

Each day you will consume:

- 1 x Sirtfood green juice
- 3 x main meals (standard or vegan options,)
- 1 to 2 x optional Sirtfood bites

Drink the juice whether in the morning, at least 30 minutes before breakfast, or in late morning.

BREAKFAST

Day 8 and 15

- Sirtfood smoothie

Day 9 and 16

- Sirt muesli

Day 10 and 17

- Yogurt with mixed berries, chopped walnuts, and dark chocolate

or

- Soy or coconut yogurt with mixed berries, chopped walnuts, and dark chocolate

Day 11 and 18

- Spiced scrambled eggs

or

- Mushroom and tofu scramble

Day 12 and 19

- Sirtfood smoothie

Day 13 and 20

- Buckwheat pancakes with strawberries, chocolate sauce, and crushed walnuts

or

- Soy or coconut yogurt with mixed berries, chopped walnuts, and dark chocolate

Day 14 and 21

- Sirtfood omelet

or

- Sirt muesli

LUNCH	DINNER
Chicken Sirt super salad	Asian shrimp stir-fry with buckwheat noodles
Waldorf salad	Tuscan bean stew
Stuffed whole-wheat pita	Butternut squash and date tagine with buckwheat
Butter bean and miso dip with celery sticks and oatcakes	Butternut squash and date tagine with buckwheat
Tuna Sirt super salad	Chicken and kale curry with Bombay potatoes
Stuffed whole-wheat pita	Kale and red onion dal with buckwheat
Strawberry buckwheat tabbouleh	Sirt chili con carne
Strawberry buckwheat tabbouleh*	Kidney bean mole with baked potato*
Waldorf salad	Smoked salmon pasta with chili and arugula
Buckwheat pasta salad	Harissa baked tofu with cauliflower "couscous"
Tofu and shiitake mushroom soup	Sirtfood pizza
Tofu and shiitake mushroom soup	Sirtfood pizza
Lentil Sirt super salad	Baked chicken breast with walnut and parsley pesto and red onion salad
Lentil Sirt super salad	Miso and sesame glazed tofu with ginger and chili stir-fried greens

After the Diet

Congrats, all Sirtfood Diet phases have now ceased! Let's just take stock of what you've actually achieved. You have reached the hyper-success process, experiencing weight loss in the region of 7 pounds which may involve some attractive growth of the muscle. During the fourteen-day maintenance process you maintained your weight loss and further improved your body composition. Above all, you've marked the beginning of your own personal health revolution. You have taken a stand against the tide of ill health which strikes as frequently as we age. The future you have chosen is greater energy, resilience and wellbeing.

We've seen why Sirtfoods are so advantageous: some plants have intricate stress-response mechanisms that generate compounds that activate sirtuins — the same fat-burning and longevity mechanism in the body that is triggered by fasting and exercise. The larger the quantity of these compounds that plants produce in response to stress, the greater the value we derive from eating them. Our majority of the best twenty Sirtfoods consists of foods that really stand out since they are particularly packed full of these compounds, and therefore the foods that have the most extraordinary ability to impact the composition and well-being of the body.

But the sirtuin-activating effects of foods aren't a whole or nothing concept. There are many other crops out there which contain moderate amounts of sirtuin-activating antioxidants and we allow you to further increase the range and diversity of your diet by consuming these liberally. The Sirtfood Diet is all about inclusion, and the better the range of sirtuin activating foods that can be added to the diet. Particularly if that means you can reap even more of your favorite food from your meals to maximize enjoyment and pleasure.

These two stages can be reworked as often as you would like to for additional weight reduction. Be that as it may, you are urged to keep eating regimen "sirtifying" after these stages have been completed by consistently consolidating sirt foods into your dinners.

There are kinds of Sirtfood Diet books filled with sirtfood-rich plans. You can also incorporate sirtfoods as a tidbit into your eating routine, or as of now you use them in plans. You're also encouraged to continue drinking the green squeeze every day.

The Sirtfood Diet thus turns out to be a way of life that changes to a greater extent than a single diet.

Chapter 6
Sirtfood Recipes

Some important notes concerning these recipes:

1. The recipes mention Thai chilies (also known as chilies with bird's eye). They are notably hotter than regular chilies if you've never had them before. If you are not used to spicy cooking, we recommend that you begin with a milder chili such as serrano, which will change the amount to suit your taste. Once you get more used to having chilies daily in your diet, you may notice that you are beginning to love hotter varieties so please do try.
2. Miso is a tasty fermented soybean paste, loaded with flavor. It comes in a variety of colors, usually white, yellow, red, and brown. The sweeter miso pastes are lighter in color than the dark ones, which can be very salty. Brown or red miso should serve well for our recipes so play with it by all measures to see which taste you like. Red

miso seems to be the saltier of these, so you will choose to use a little less of it if you go for this one. Miso 's flavor and saltiness can also vary from product to product, so the best option would be to verify which kinds you buy and change the level you use appropriately, so it isn't too intoxicating. That requires a bit of trial and error, but eventually you'll get the best of it.

3. It couldn't be better if you haven't eaten buckwheat yet. We suggest that you rinse the buckwheat vigorously in a sieve first before putting it into a saucepan of hot water. Baking times can vary so verify your bundle guidelines.

4. It would be better for all the meals to have flat-leaf parsley, but if you can't make sense of it, frizzy it will.

5. Onions, garlic, and ginger shall always be removed unless stated otherwise.

6. These recipes do not use salt and pepper, but feel free to season with sea salt and black pepper to suit your own personal tastes. Sirtfoods deliver so much flavor, you'll actually find that you don't need as many as you usually do. It is strongly suggested to apply black pepper to any dish that includes turmeric, because this will further improve the absorption of the main sirtuin-activating compound, curcumin.

Asian Shrimp Stir-Fry with Buckwheat Noodles

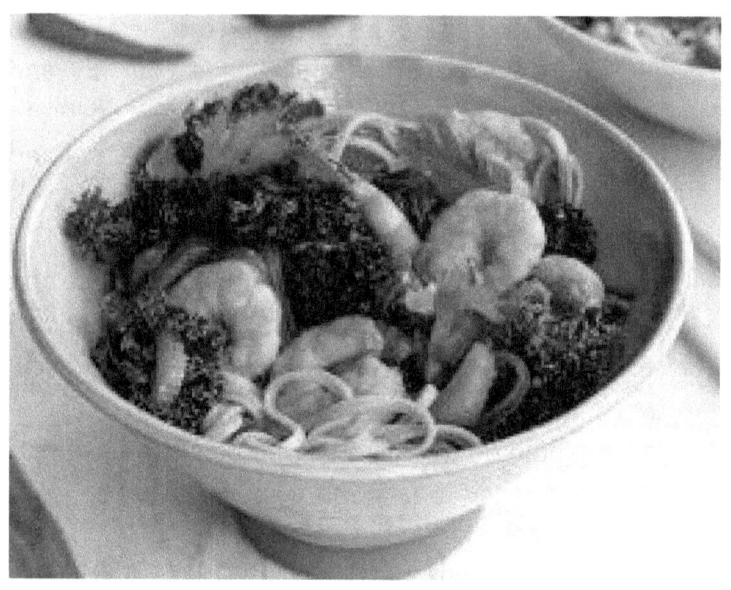

Ingredients	Quantity
Shelled raw jumbo shrimp, deveined	1/3 pound (150g)
Tamari (or soy sauce if you are not avoiding gluten)	2 teaspoons
Extra virgin olive oil	2 teaspoons
Soba (buckwheat noodles)	3 ounces (75g)
Garlic cloves, finely sliced	2
Thai chili, finely sliced	1
Teaspoon finely sliced fresh ginger	1
Red onions, sliced	1/8 cup (20g)
Celery including leaves, trimmed,	1/2 cup (45g)

and sliced, with leaves set aside
Green beans, chopped — 1/2 cup (75g)
Kale, roughly chopped — 3/4 cup (50g)
Chicken stock — 1/2 cup (100ml)

SERVES 1

INSTRUCTIONS

1. Steam a deep fryer over high temperature, then cook the shrimp for two or three minutes in 1 tablespoon tamari and one teaspoon oil. Put the shrimp into a tray. Flush the skillet out with a towel of paper, as you will be using it again.
2. Bake the noodles for five to eight minutes in boiling water, or as indicated on the box. Flush and put away.
3. Elsewhere, in the leftover tamari and oil over medium-high heat, cook the garlic, ginger, chili, celery, red onion, (but not the leaves), kale and green beans for two to three min. Remove the stocks and bring to a simmer, then steam for a couple of minutes until baked and yet crunchy.
4. Add the shrimp, pasta, and foliage of celery to the bowl, bring to a simmer, turn off the heat and drink.

Miso and Sesame Glazed Tofu with Ginger and Chili Stir-Fried Greens

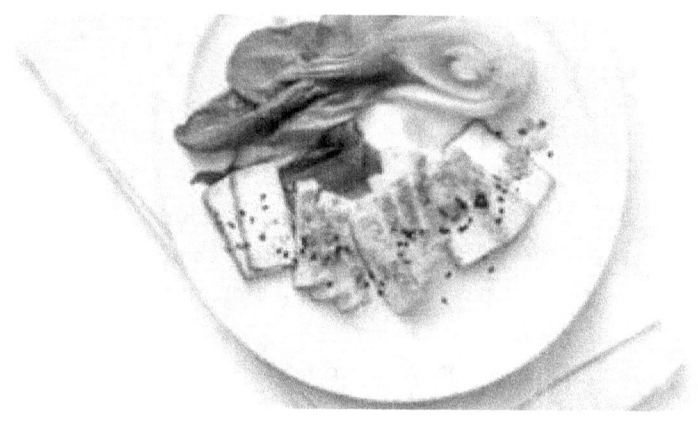

Ingredients	Quantity
Mirin	1 tablespoon
Miso paste	3 $^{1/2}$ teaspoons (20g)
Block of rm tofu	1 x 5-ounce (150g)
Celery, trimmed (about 1/3 cup when sliced)	1 stalk (40g)
Red onion, sliced	1/4 cup (40g)
Zucchini (about 1 cup when sliced)	1 small (120g)
Thai chili	1
Garlic cloves	2
Teaspoon finely sliced fresh ginger	1
Kale, chopped	3/4 cup (50g)

Sesame seeds	2 teaspoons
Buckwheat	1/4 cup (35g)
Ground turmeric	1 teaspoon
Extra virgin olive oil	2 teaspoons
Tamari (or soy sauce if you are not avoiding gluten)	1 teaspoon

SERVES 1

INSTRUCTIONS

1. Heat oven up to 400oF (200oC). Line a thin, parchment-paper baking dish.
2. Blend both the mirin and the miso. Lengthwise cut the tofu, then diagonal direction split each slice into triangle in half. Wrap the tofu with the miso blending and allow to marinate while the other items are packed.
3. Chop the direction into the celery and red onion. Chop the chili, garlic, and ginger thinly, and cast aside.
4. Heat the Kale for five minutes in a container. Discard and put back.
5. Spot the tofu in the baking dish, stir the tofu with the sesame seeds and bake in the oven for fifteen to twenty minutes until it has been beautifully caramelized.
6. Wipe the buckwheat in a mesh, then put this along with the turmeric in a saucepan of boiling hot water. Process as indicated by box, then rinse. Steam the oil in a saucepan; introduce the onion, celery, zucchini, chili, garlic and ginger

and fry over high heat for one to two minutes, then decrease to moderate flame for approximately 3 minutes until the vegetables are baked through yet are crunchy. If the vegetables start sticking to the skillet you may have to append a spoonful of water. Attach the tamari and kale and cook for 1 minute.
7. Represent with the leaves and buckwheat when the tofu is set.

Turkey Escalope with Sage, Capers, Parsley and Spiced Cauliflower Couscous

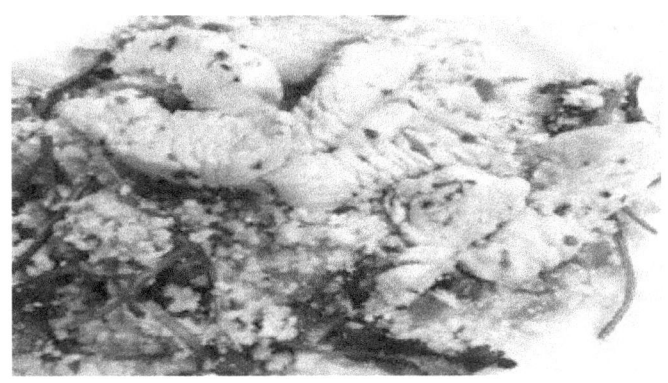

Slender cutlets are great but there are two best ways to turn it into an escalope if you can only figure turkey breast. You should either use a meat tenderizer, a spike, or a rolling pin to beat the steak until it becomes around 1/4 inch (5 mm) thick, based on how dense the chest is. Alternatively, if you find like the chest is too hard to deal with, and you have a strong hand, split the chest half horizontally and strike each section with the tenderizer.

Ingredients	*Quantity*
Cauliflower, roughly chopped	1 $^{1/2}$ cups (150g)
Garlic cloves, finely sliced	2
Red onion, finely sliced	1/4 cup (40g)
Thai chili, finely sliced	1
Finely sliced fresh ginger	1 teaspoon
Extra virgin olive oil	2 tablespoons
Ground turmeric	2 teaspoons
Sun-dried tomatoes, finely sliced	1/2 cup (30g)

Fresh parsley, chopped	1/4 cup (10g)
Turkey cutlet or steak (see above)	1/3-pound (150g)
Dried sage	1 teaspoon
Juice of lemon	¼
Capers	1 tablespoon

SERVES 1

INSTRUCTIONS

1. Put the raw cabbage in a mixing bowl to produce the "couscous" Pulse to thinly slice the cabbage in 2-second flashes until it mimics a couscous. Conversely, you should use a razor, then finely sliced it.
2. In 1 tablespoon of the oil, cook the red onion, garlic, chili, and ginger unless it is soft but not browned. Insert the cabbage and turmeric and continue cooking for one minute. Remove the tomatoes from pan and add half of the parsley.
3. Cover the meat escalope in the herb and just a little butter, then cook in a large skillet over medium heat for four to six minutes using residual oil, turning periodically. Add the lemon juice, residual parsley, capers and 1 tablespoon of water to the skillet when fried across. This should make a cabbage sauce to drink.

Kale and Red Onion Dal with Buckwheat

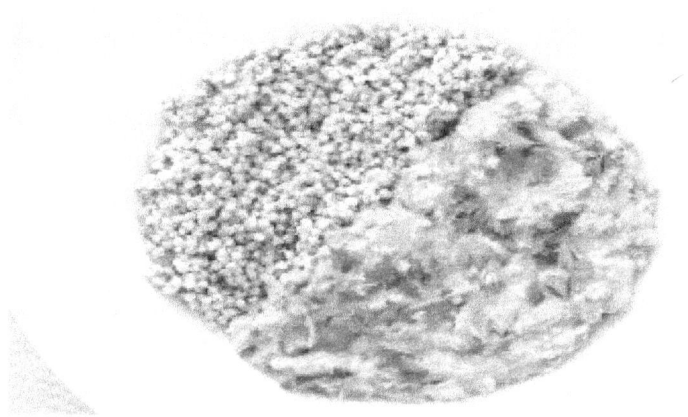

Ingredients	Quantity
Extra virgin olive oil	1 teaspoon
Mustard seeds	1 teaspoon
Red onion, finely sliced	1/4 cup (40g)
Garlic cloves, finely sliced	2
Finely sliced fresh ginger	1 teaspoon
Thai chili, finely sliced	1
Mild curry powder (medium or hot if you prefer)	1 teaspoon
Ground turmeric	2 teaspoons
Vegetable stock or water	1 1/4 cups (300ml)
Red lentils, rinsed	1/4 cup (40g)
Kale, chopped	3/4 cup (50g)
Tinned coconut milk	3 1/2 tablespoons (50ml)
Buckwheat	1/3 cup (50g)

SERVES 1

INSTRUCTIONS

1. Heat the oil over moderate flame in a small saucepan and bring the mustard seeds. When the mustard seeds begin popping, introduce the onion, ginger, garlic, and chili. Fry until smooth, for about ten minutes.
2. Add the turmeric curry powder and one tablespoon, then steam the seasoning for a few minutes. Stir in the stock and bring to a simmer. Attach the lentils to the saucepan and boil for another twenty-five to thirty minutes before the lentils are fried through and a glossy dal is available.
3. Start adding milk to the kale and coconut and bake for another five minutes.
4. In the meantime, fry the buckwheat with the leftover turmeric tablespoon, as per the box guidance. Flush and eat with the dal.

Aromatic Chicken Breast with Kale Red Onions, and Tomato and Chili Salsa

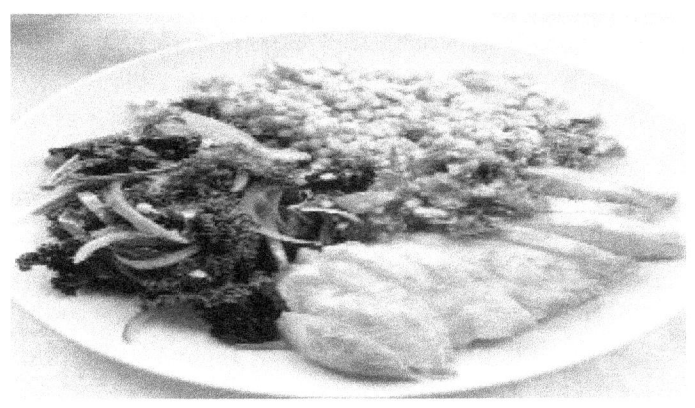

Ingredients	Quantity
Skinless, boneless chicken breast	1/4 pound (120g)
Ground turmeric	2 teaspoons
Juice of lemon	¼
Extra-virgin olive oil	1 tablespoon
Kale, chopped	3/4 cup (50g)
Red onion, sliced	1/8 cup (20g)
Chopped fresh ginger	1 teaspoon
Buckwheat	1/3 cup (50g)
FOR THE SALSA	
Medium tomato	1 of (130g)
Thai chili, finely sliced	1
Capers, finely sliced	1 tablespoon
Parsley, finely sliced	2 tablespoons (5g)
Juice of lemon	¼

SERVES 1

INSTRUCTIONS

1. Start by removing the eye from the tomato to make the salsa, and slicing it quite well, trying to take care to keep as much of the fluid as feasible. Blend with the chili, parsley, capers, and lemon juice. You might put it all in a mixer, but the final outcome is a little distinct.
2. Heat the oven up to 220 ° C (425oF). In one teaspoon of turmeric, the lemon juice, and a little oil, marinate the roast chicken. Turn on for five to ten minutes.
3. Steam an oven-proof deep fryer until warm, then introduce the marinated chicken and roast on each side for about a moment or so until pale golden, then switch to the oven (set on a cookie sheet if your skillet is not oven-proof) for eight to ten minutes or till roasted. Remove from heat, wrap in foil, then leave for five minutes to relax before having to serve.
4. In the meantime, boil the kale for five minutes in a container. Cook the red onions and the ginger in that little oil, then add the cooked kale and cook for the next moment till smooth but not golden brown.
5. Fry the buckwheat with the residual turmeric tablespoon, as per package directions. Serve with meat, leafy greens, and salsa.

HARISSA BAKED TOFU WITH CAULIFLOWER "COUSCOUS"

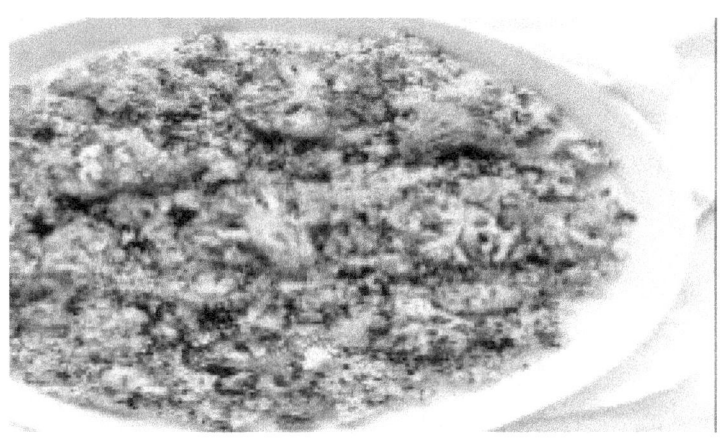

Ingredients	Quantity
Red bell pepper	3/8 cup (60g)
Thai chili, cut in half	1
Garlic cloves	2
Extra-virgin olive oil	about 1 tablespoon
Ground cumin	pinch of
Ground coriander	pinch of
Juice of lemon	¼
Rm tofu	7 ounces (200g)
Cauliflower, roughly chopped	1 ¾ cups (200g)
Red onion, finely sliced	1/4 cup (40g)
Finely sliced fresh ginger	1 teaspoon
Ground turmeric	2 teaspoons
Sun-dried tomatoes, finely sliced	1/2 cup (30g)
Parsley, chopped	1/2 cup (20g)

SERVES 1

INSTRUCTIONS

1. Heat the oven to 400ºF (200ºC).
2. Chop the red pepper elongated from around center to make the harissa so you have good pieces, erase any seeds, after which spot the chili and one of the garlic cloves in a baking dish. Add a little oil and the thawed cumin and coriander and fry for fifteen to twenty minutes in the oven till the peppers are smooth but not too gray. With oven on at this setting mix with the lemon juice into a mixing bowl till light and fluffy.
3. Lengthwise chunk the tofu and then in the diagonal direction cut into triangles each half. Spot in a small detachable casserole dish or one lined with baking parchment, replace with harissa and grill for twenty minutes in the oven — the tofu should have consumed the marinade and started turning dark red.
4. To make the "couscous," put the raw cauliflower in a meal
5. Pulse to thinly slice the cabbage in 2-second flashes till it mimics a couscous. Conversely, you can use a blade, and thinly slice it.
6. Strip out the last clove of garlic. In one tablespoon of oil, roast the ginger, red onion, and garlic, until softened but not golden brown, then introduce the turmeric and cabbage and cook over medium heat for one minute.
7. Remove from heat and mix in the tomatoes and parsley, which are dried with light. Serve with the tofu which is fried.

Sirt Muesli

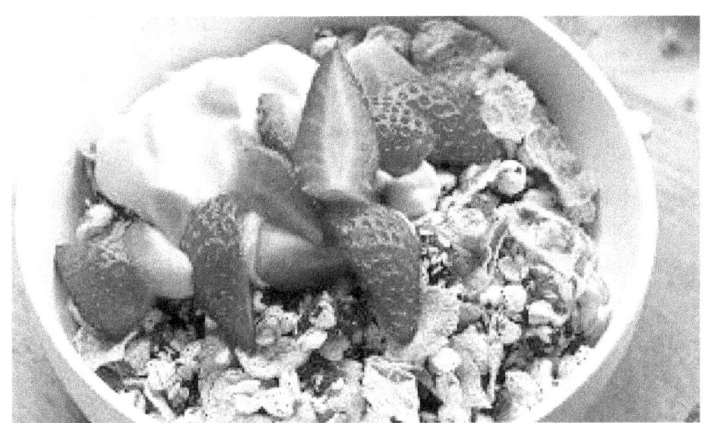

You just combine the dry ingredients and put the combination in an enclosed jar if you want to make this in abundance or cook it the evening before. The very next day all you have to do is introduce the strawberries and milk and it's ready to go.

Ingredients	Quantity
Buckwheat flakes	1/4 cup (20g)
Buckwheat puffs	2/3 cup (10g)
Coconut flakes or dried coconut	3 tablespoons (15g)
Medjool dates, pitted and chopped	1/4 cup (40g)
Walnuts, chopped	1/8 cup (15g)
Cocoa nibs	1 1/2 tablespoons

	(10g)
Strawberries, hulled and chopped	2/3 cup (100g)
Plain Greek yogurt (or vegan alternative, such as soy or coconut yogurt)	3/8 cup (100g)

SERVES 1

INSTRUCTIONS

1. Mix all of the ingredients together (leave out the strawberries and yogurt if not serving right away).

Pan-Fried Salmon Fillet With Caramelized Endive, Arugula, and Cherry Leaf Salad

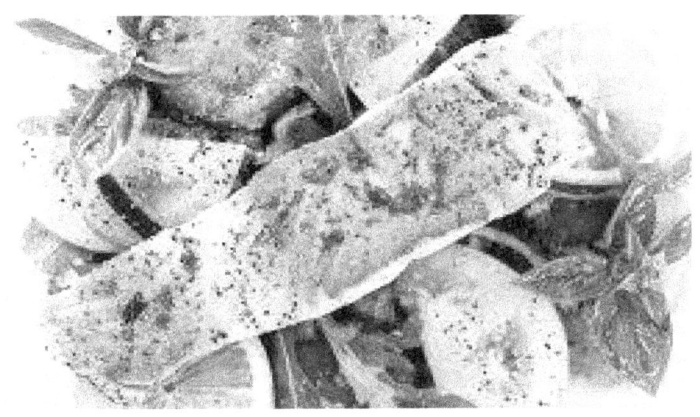

Ingredients	Quantity
Parsley	1/4 cup (10g)
Juice of lemon	¼
Capers	1 tablespoon
Clove garlic, roughly chopped	1
Extra-virgin olive oil	1 tablespoon
Avocado, peeled, stoned, and diced	1/4
Cherry tomatoes, cut in half	2/3 cup (100g)
Red onion, thinly sliced	1/8 cup (20g)
Arugula	1 3/4 ounces (50g)
Celery leaves	2 tablespoons (5g)
Skinless salmon fillet	1 x 5-ounce (150g)
Brown sugar	2 teaspoons
Head of endive (1), cut in half lengthways	about 2 1/2 ounces (70g)

SERVES 1

INSTRUCTIONS

1. Heat the oven up to 220 ° C (425oF).
2. Put the parsley, garlic, lemon juice, capers, and two teaspoons of oil in a mixing bowl or blender for dressing and mix until thick and creamy.
3. For the salad, combine the leaves of red onion, tomato, arugula, avocado and celery.
4. Warm a frying casserole over high temperature. Massage the salmon in a little oil and sear for a moment or so in the frying skillet to caramelize the exterior. Exchange to a small bowl and bake in the oven for four to six minutes or until it is finished cooking; decrease the heating process by two minutes if you like the pink presented inside of your fish.
5. Wash the saucepan out afterwards and put everything back on high fire. Mix the brown sugar with the remaining oil teaspoon and sprinkle it over the endive cut sides. Position the sides of the endive cut into the skillet and cook for two or three minutes, trying to turn frequently, until tender and perfectly golden brown. In the sauce, mix the salad and top with tuna, and endive.

Tuscan Bean Stew

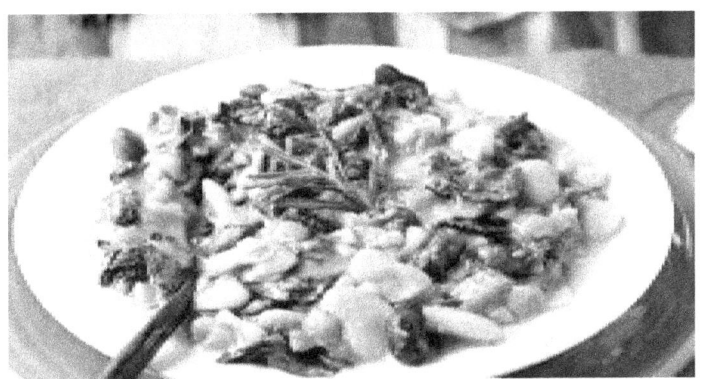

Ingredients	Quantity
Extra-virgin olive oil	1 tablespoon
Red onion, finely chopped	1/3 cup (50g)
Carrot, peeled and finely sliced	1/4 cup (30g)
Celery, trimmed and finely sliced	1/3 cup (30g)
Garlic cloves, finely sliced	2
Thai chili, finely sliced (optional)	1/2
Herbs de Provence	1 teaspoon
Vegetuble stock	7/8 cup (200ml)
Chopped Italian tomatoes	1 x 14-ounce can (400g)
Tomato purée	1 teaspoon
Canned mixed beans (drained weight)	3/4 cup (130g)
Kale, roughly chopped	3/4 cup (50g)
Roughly chopped parsley	1 tablespoon
Buckwheat	1/4 cup (40g)

SERVES 1

INSTRUCTIONS

1. Consider placing the oil over low to moderate heat in a small saucepan and cook the onion, garlic, carrot, celery, chili (if used) and herb carefully, till the onion becomes softer but not golden brown.
2. Stir in the tomatoes, stock, and purée tomatoes and bring to a simmer. Bring the beans and allow to cook for thirty min.
3. Bring the kale and prepare food for the next five to ten minutes, then introduce the parsley, till bidding process.
4. In the meantime, as per the official guidelines, fry the buckwheat, flush, and then start serving with the stew.

Strawberry Buckwheat Tabbouleh

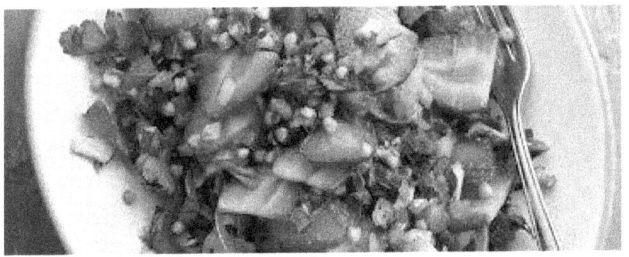

Ingredients	Quantity
Buckwheat	1/3 cup (50g)
Ground turmeric	1 tablespoon
Avocado	1/2 cup (80g)
Tomato	3/8 cup (65g)
Red onion	1/8 cup (20g)
Medjool dates, pitted	1/8 cup (25g)
Capers	1 tablespoon
Parsley	3/4 cup (30g)
Strawberries, hulled	2/3 cup (100g)
Extra-virgin olive oil	1 tablespoon
Juice of lemon	½
Arugula	1-ounce (30g)

SERVES 1

INSTRUCTIONS

1. Process the buckwheat with the turmeric as indicated on the box. Sink to chill and set it aside.
2. Start cutting the avocado, basil, red onion, capers, dates, and parsley thinly and blend with the fresh buckwheat. Pick the strawberries, then blend the oil then lemon juice softly into the dish. Represent on an earthenware bed.

Miso-Marinated Baked Cod with Stir-Fried Greens and Sesame

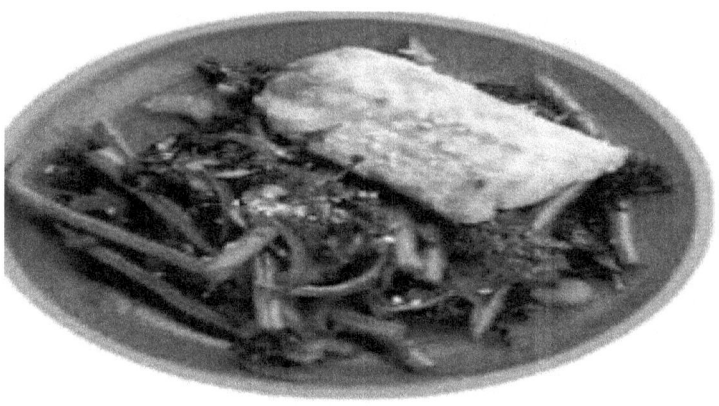

Ingredients	Quantity
Miso	3 1/2 teaspoons (20g)
Mirin	1 tablespoon
Extra-virgin olive oil	1 tablespoon
Skinless cod fillet	1 x 7-ounce (200g)
Red onion, sliced	1/8 cup (20g)
Celery, sliced	3/8 cup (40g)
Garlic cloves, finely sliced	2
Thai chili, finely sliced	1
Finely sliced fresh ginger	1 teaspoon
Green beans	3/8 cup (60g)
Kale, roughly chopped	3/4 cup (50g)
Sesame seeds	1 teaspoon
Parsley, roughly chopped	2 tablespoons (5g)
Tamari (or soy sauce if	1 tablespoon

you are not avoiding gluten)	
Buckwheat	1/4 cup (40g)
Ground turmeric	1 teaspoon

SERVES 1

INSTRUCTIONS

1. Blend the oil with the mirin, miso and 1 teaspoon. Massage the cod all over and consider leaving for thirty min to marinate. Heat the oven up to 220 ° C (425oF).
2. Cook the cod for ten minutes.
3. In the meantime, heat the residual oil to a large skillet or wok. Stir-fry the onion for another few minutes, then bring the celery, chili, garlic, ginger, green beans, and kale. Toss and roast till the kale is roasted through and crispy. To help the frying process you might have to bring a little water to the skillet.
4. Fry the buckwheat along with the turmeric as per the manufacturer's guidelines.
5. To the stir-fry insert the parsley, sesame seeds, and tamari and represent with buckwheat and salmon.

Soba (Buckwheat Noodles) in a Miso Broth with Tofu, Celery, and Kale

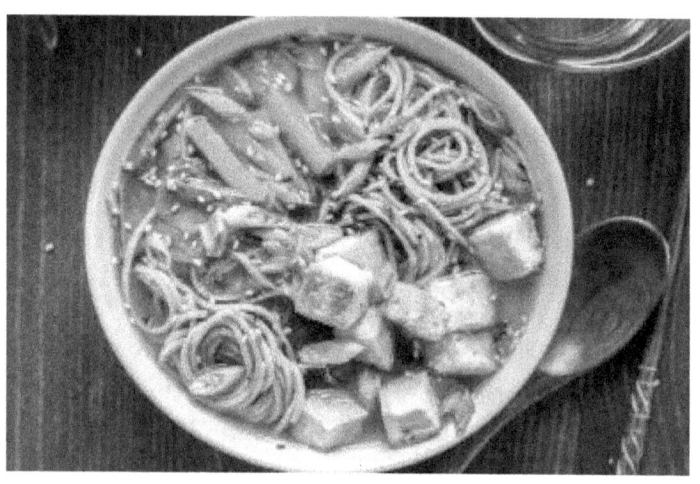

Ingredients	Quantity
Soba (buckwheat noodles)	3 ounces (75g)
Extra-virgin olive oil	1 tablespoon
Red onion, sliced	1/8 cup (20g)
Garlic cloves, finely sliced	2
Finely sliced fresh ginger	1 teaspoon
Vegetable stock, plus a little extra, if necessary	1 1/4 cups (300ml)
Miso paste	1 3/4 tablespoons (30g)
Kale, roughly chopped	3/4 cup (50g)
Celery, roughly chopped	1/2 cup (50g)
Sesame seeds	1 teaspoon

Rm tofu, cut into ¼ - to ½ - inch (0.5 to 1cm) cubes (about 3/8 cup)	3 1/2 ounces (100g)
Tamari (optional; or soy sauce if you are not avoiding gluten)	1 teaspoon

SERVES 1

INSTRUCTIONS

1. Put the noodles in a saucepan of hot water and cook for five to eight minutes or as indicated on the box.
2. In a frying pan, start adding the oil; add the garlic, onions, ginger, and fry in the oil over moderate flame until tender, but not golden brown. Stir in stocks and miso and put to a simmer.
3. Bring the kale and celery to the miso broth and cook delicately for five min (try not to heat up the miso as you demolish the taste and make it textured smudgy). As needed, you might need to append a little more stock.
4. Insert the fried noodles and sesame seeds and permit the tofu to heat up. If needed, start serving in a bowl slathered with some tamari.

Sirt Super Salad

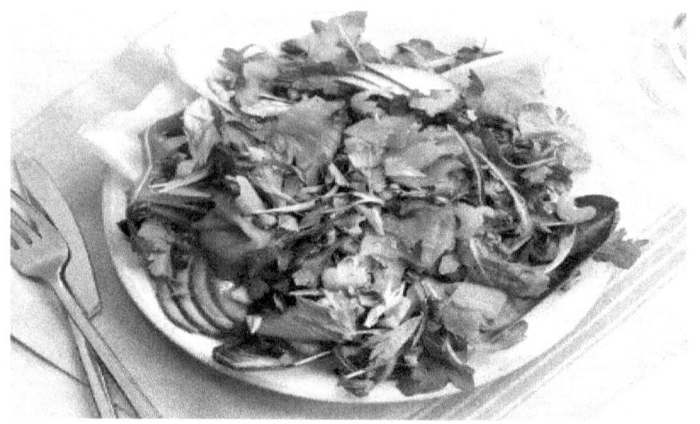

Ingredients	Quantity
Arugula	1 3/4 ounces (50g)
Endive leaves	1 3/4 ounces (50g)
Smoked salmon slices	3 1/2 ounces (100g)
Avocado, peeled, stoned, and sliced	1/2 cup (80g)
Celery including leaves, sliced	1/2 cup (50g)
Red onion, sliced	1/8 cup (20g)
Walnuts, chopped	1/8 cups (15g)
Capers	1 tablespoon
Large Medjool date, pitted and chopped	1
Extra-virgin olive oil	1 tablespoon
Juice of lemon	¼
Parsley, chopped	1/4 cup (10g)

SERVES 1

INSTRUCTIONS

1. Position the leaf of salad on a tray, or in a plastic bucket. Blend all the rest of the ingredients and represent over the foliage.

VARIATIONS

1. Substitute the roasted salmon with 11/3 cups (100 g) canned green lentils or grilled Le Puy lentils for a **lentil** Sirt super salad.
2. Start replacing the roasted salmon with a chopped cooked chicken chest, for a **chicken** Sirt fantastic salad.
3. Start replacing the roasted salmon with canned tuna for a **tuna** Sirt super salad (in oil or water, as preferred).

Char-Grilled Beef with a Red Wine Jus, Onion Rings, Garlic Kale, and Herb-Roasted Potatoes

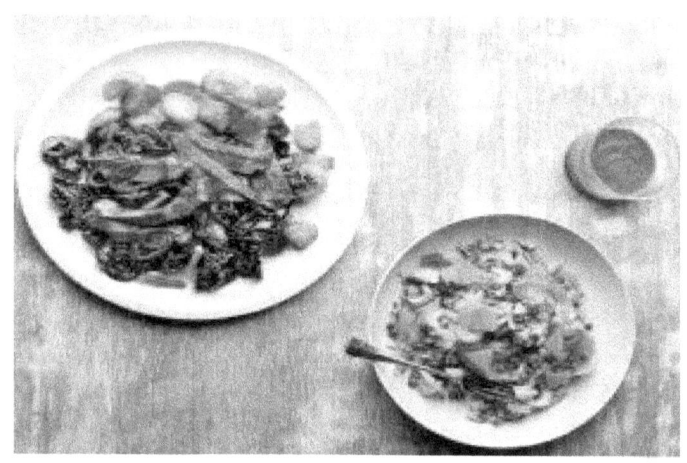

Ingredients	Quantity
Potatoes, peeled and cut into Diced pieces	1/2 cup (100g) 3/4-inch (2cm)
Extra-virgin olive oil	1 tablespoon
Parsley, finely sliced	2 tablespoons (5g)
Red onion, sliced into rings	1/3 cup (50g)
Kale, sliced	2 ounces (50g)
Garlic cloves, finely sliced	2
Beef tenderloin (about 1 ½ inches or 3.5cm thick) or sirloin steak (¾ inch or 2cm thick)	1 x 4- to 5-ounce (120 to 150g)
Red wine	3 tablespoons (40ml)
Beef stock	5/8 cup (150ml)
Tomato purée	1 teaspoon
Corn our, dissolved in 1 tablespoon water	1 teaspoon

SERVES 1

INSTRUCTIONS

1. Heat the oven up to 425ºF (220ºC). Put the potatoes in a hot water frying pan, bring them back to a simmer and prepare food for four to five minutes, then wash. Put one teaspoon of oil in a large skillet and cook for thirty-five to forty minutes in the preheated oven. Flip the potatoes every ten minutes to make sure baking is even done. Remove from heat when finished, spray with the minced garlic and stir well.
2. Cook the onion over moderate flame in one teaspoon of the oil for approximately five minutes, until it is smooth and crispy. Hold on warm.
3. Heat the kale for two to three minutes, then wash. In 1/2 teaspoon of oil, cook the garlic softly for one minute, till thin but not gray. Insert the kale and cook for another one to two minutes, till soft. Hold on warm.
4. Warm up a frying pan which is ovenproof over high temperature before burned. Wrap the meat with 1/2 teaspoon of oil and roast over moderate to high heat in the frying skillet, depending on how much you like your meat (see our baking time guidance). If you like your meat medium, it would be best to caramelize it and then move it to an oven set at 425oF (220oC) for the specified times.
5. Take the meat from the saucepan and laid to rest. To bring up any meat remaining add the wine to the skillet. Boil to halve the wine, until it

becomes fizzy and has a high concentration flavor.
6. Add the dry ingredients and tomato purée to the steak skillet and bring to a simmer, then introduce the corn-our paste to firm up your recipe, trying to add it slightly at a moment till the required consistency is reached. Add any of the rested steak juices, and start serving with the fried potatoes, kale, onion rings, and wine sauce.

Steak Cooking Times

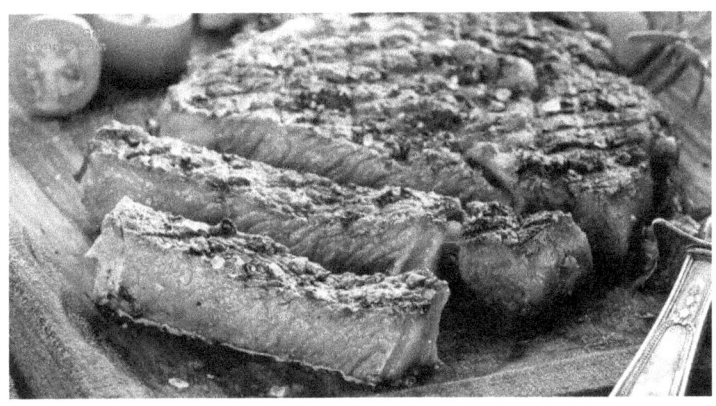

Ingredients	Quantity
TENDERLOIN	1$^{1/2}$-INCH-THICK (3.5CM)
Blue	about 1 $^{1/2}$ minutes each side
Rare	about 2 $^{1/4}$ minutes each side
Medium-rare	about 3 $^{1/4}$ minutes each side
Medium	about 4 $^{1/2}$ minutes each side
SIRLOIN STEAK	**3/4-INCH-THICK (2CM)**
Blue	about 1 minute each side
Rare	about 1 $^{1/2}$ minutes each side
Medium-rare	about 2 minutes each side
Medium	about 2 $^{1/4}$ minutes each side

Kidney Bean Mole with Baked Potato

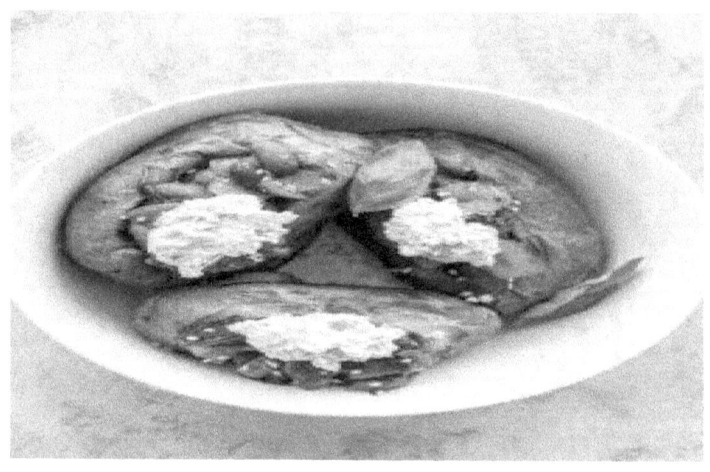

Ingredients	Quantity
Red onion, finely sliced	1/4 cup (40g)
Fnely sliced fresh ginger	1 teaspoon
giarlic cloves, finely sliced	2
Thai chili, finely sliced	1
Teaspoon extra virgin olive oil	1
Ground turmeric	1 teaspoon
Ground cumin	1 teaspoon
Ground clove	pinch of
Ground cinnamon	pinch of
Medium baking potato	1
Canned chopped tomatoes	7/8 cup (190g)
Brown sugar	1 teaspoon
Red bell pepper, cored, seeds removed, and roughly chopped	1/3 cup (50g)
Vegetable stock	5/8 cup (150ml)
Cocoa powder	1 tablespoon
Sesame seeds	1 teaspoon

Peanut butter (smooth if available, but chunky is ne)	2 teaspoons
Canned kidney beans	7/8 cup (150g)
Parsley, chopped	2 tablespoons (5g)

SERVES 1

INSTRUCTIONS

1. Heat the oven up to 400°F (200ºC).
2. In a small saucepan, cook the onion, garlic, ginger, and chili in the oil over moderate flame for about ten minutes, until its soft. Add the ingredients and continue cooking for one to two more minutes.
3. Put the potato on a cookie sheet in the heated pan and roast until smooth in the midpoint (or largely dependent on how caramelized you like the outside) for forty-five to fifty minutes.
4. In the meantime, add to the casserole the sugar, tomatoes, red pepper, stock, peanut butter, cocoa powder, sesame seeds, and kidney beans and cook lightly for forty-five to sixty minutes.
5. At the end spray with the parsley. Sliced the potato in half, then start serving the mole over it.

Sirtfood Omelet

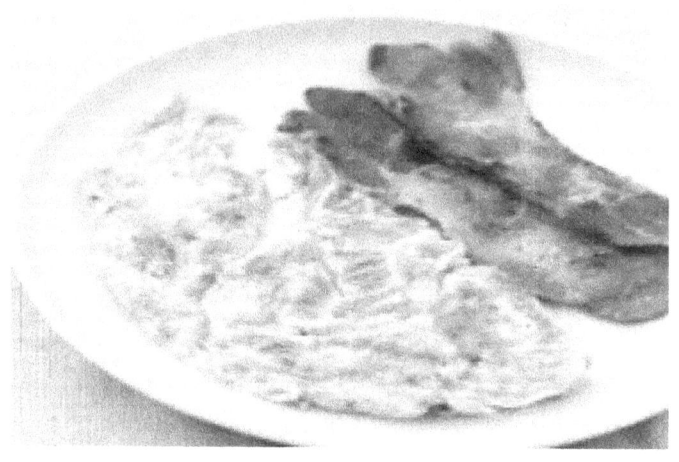

Ingredients	Quantity
Sliced streaky bacon (or 2 rashers, smoked or regular, depending on your taste)	about 2 ounces (50g)
Medium eggs	3
Red endive, thinly sliced	1 1/4 ounces (35g)
Parsley, finely sliced	2 tablespoons (5g)
Turmeric	1 teaspoon
Extra virgin olive oil	1 teaspoon

SERVES 1

INSTRUCTIONS

1. Heat up a deep fryer with a nonstick. Chopped the bacon into small slices, and roast until toasty, over high temperature. You shouldn't need to append oil the bacon contains sufficient fat for cooking. Remove from heat and put any extra fat

on a clean cloth. Flush clean cup.
2. Beat the eggs and blend the endive, the parsley as well as the turmeric together. Cut the steamed bacon into squares and mix in the eggs.
3. In the cooking pot, warm the oil-the pan must be warm but not smoking. Append the egg mixture and relocate it around the pan using a spatula to actually cook the egg. Retain the fried egg bits moving and rotate around the bowl till the omelet amount is even. Decrease fire and encourage the omelet to cook a bit more. Relieve the spatula around the corners and flip in half the omelet or slide up and serve.

Baked Chicken Breast with Walnut and Parsley Pesto and Red Onion Salad

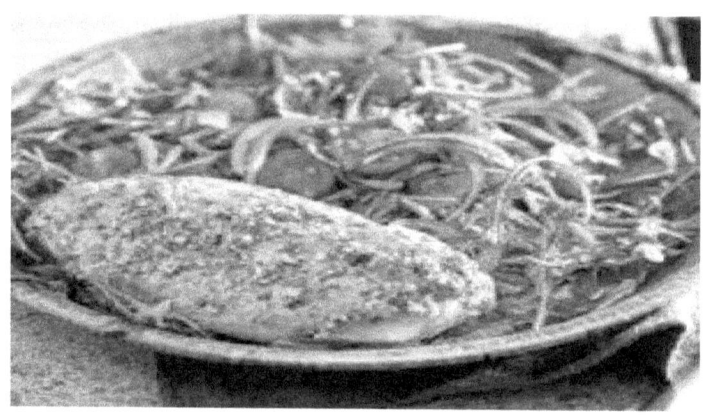

Ingredients	Quantity
Parsley	3/8 cup (15g)
Walnuts	1/8 cup (15g)
Parmesan cheese, grated	4 teaspoons (15g)
Extra-virgin olive oil	1 tablespoon
Juice of lemon	½
Water	3 tablespoons (50ml)
Skinless chicken breast	5 1/2 ounces (150g)
Red onions, finely sliced	1/8 cup (20g)
Red wine vinegar	1 teaspoon
Arugula	1 1/4 ounces (35g)
Cherry tomatoes, cut in half	2/3 cup (100g)
Balsamic vinegar	1 teaspoon

SERVES 1

INSTRUCTIONS

1. To prepare the pesto, put the parsley, parmesan, walnuts, olive oil, a little amount of the lemon juice, and some water in a skillet or blender and mix unless a smooth paste is in place. Progressively append more water before you have the quality you want.
2. In the refrigerator, caramelize the roast chicken in one tablespoon of pesto and the residual lemon juice for thirty min, for longer time if feasible.
3. Preheat the oven up to 400ºF (200ºC).
4. Warm a deep fryer which is ovenproof over moderate to high heat. In its marinade, roast the chicken from either edge for one minute, then move the saucepan to the oven to bake for eight minutes or till roasted.
5. Caramelize the onions for five to ten minutes in a red wine vinegar. Flush fluid.
6. So, if roasted, remove the chicken from the heat, spoon another tablespoon of pesto through it, and then let the chicken warmth dissolve the pesto. Wrap in foil and risk leaving for five min to settle before representing.
7. Merge the balsamic vinegar with the tomatoes, arugula, and onion and drizzle. Represent with the meat and spoon over the pesto left over.

Waldorf Salad

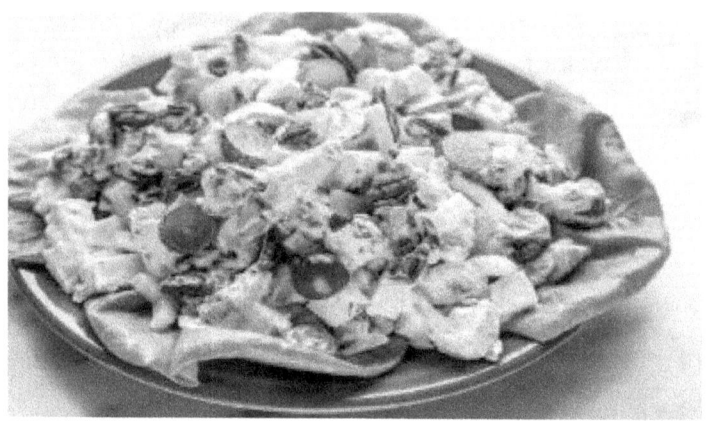

Ingredients	Quantity
Celery including leaves, roughly chopped	1 cup (100g)
Apple, roughly chopped	1/2 cup (50g)
Walnuts, roughly chopped	3/8 cup (50g)
Red onion, roughly chopped	1 tablespoon (10g)
Parsley, chopped	2 tablespoons (5g)
Capers	1 tablespoon
Extra-virgin olive oil	1 tablespoon
Balsamic vinegar	1 teaspoon
Juice of lemon	¼
Dijon mustard	1/4 teaspoon
Arugula	about 2 ounces (50g)
Endive leaves	about 1 1/2 ounces (35g)

SERVES 1

INSTRUCTIONS

1. Blend with the parsley and capers, the celery and its foliage, onion, walnuts, and apple.
2. To prepare the dressing whisk the vinegar, oil, lemon juice and mustard in a pan.
3. Start serving the combination of celery on top of the rug and endive with the coating and spill over it

Roasted Eggplant Wedges with Walnut and Parsley Pesto and Tomato Salad

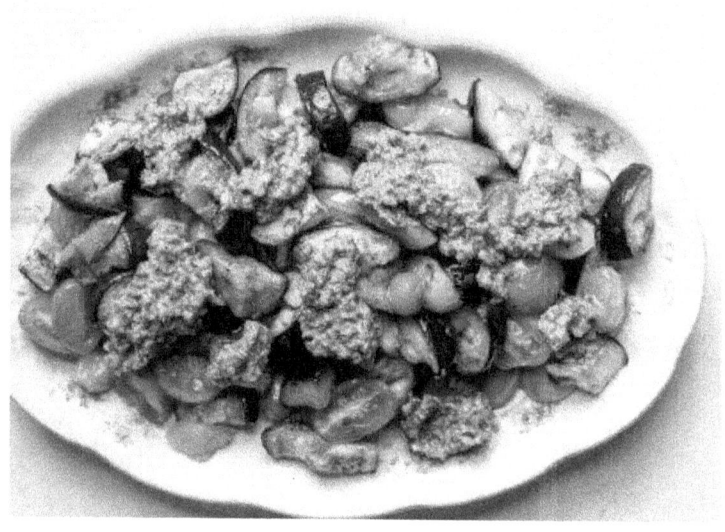

Ingredients	Quantity
Parsley	1/2 cup (20g)
Walnuts	3/4 ounces (20g)
Parmesan cheese (or use a vegetarian or vegan alternative), grated	1/8 cup (20g)
Extra-virgin olive oil	1 tablespoon
Juice of lemon	¼
Water	3 tablespoons (50ml)
Eggplant, quartered	1 small (around 5 1/2 ounces or 150g)

Red onions, sliced	1/8 cup (20g)
Red wine vinegar	1 teaspoon (5ml)
Arugula	1 1/4 ounces (35g)
Cherry tomatoes	2/3 cup (100g)
Balsamic vinegar	1 teaspoon (5ml)

SERVES 1

INSTRUCTIONS

1. Heat the oven up to 400ºF (200ºC).
2. Put the parsley, walnuts, parmesan, olive oil and quarter the lemon juice in a mixing bowl or mixer to start making the pesto and mix and you'll have a fine consistency. Progressively insert the water till you have the good consistency — this should be dense enough for the eggplant to adhere to.
3. Spray the eggplant with some pesto and reserve the remainder to start serving. Put on a cookie sheet and grill for twenty-five to thirty minutes, till the gray, smooth, and soggy eggplant is golden.
4. In the meantime, coat with the red wine vinegar over through the red onion and cast aside — this should smooth and caramelize the onion. Flush the vinegar and serve.
5. Merge the arugula, tomatoes, and flush the onion and sprinkle the salad over the balsamic vinegar. Start serving with soft eggplant, squishing over the leftover pesto.

Sirtfood Smoothie

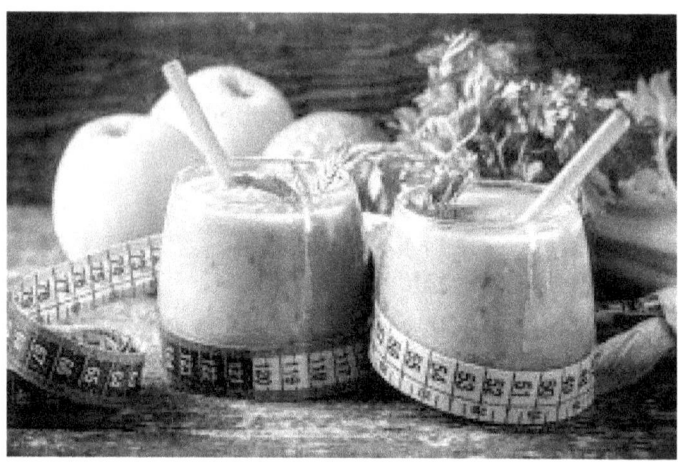

Ingredients	Quantity
plain Greek yogurt (or vegan alternative, such as soy or coconut yogurt)	3/8 cup (100g)
walnut halves	6
strawberries, hulled	8 to 10 medium size
handful of kale, stalks removed	
dark chocolate (85 percent cocoa solids)	3/4 ounce (20g)
Medjool date, pitted	1
ground turmeric	1/2 teaspoon
thin sliver of Thai chili	(1 to 2mm)
unsweetened almond milk	7/8 cup (200ml)

SERVES 1

INSTRUCTIONS

1. In a food processor, rumble ingredients until bouncy and light.

Stuffed Whole-Wheat Pita

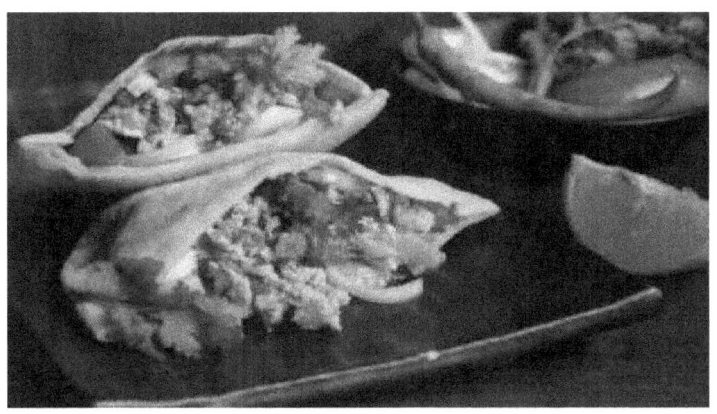

Ingredients	Quantity
FOR A MEAT OPTION	
Cooked turkey slices, chopped	3 ounces (80g)
Cheddar cheese, diced	3/4-ounce (20g)
Cucumber, diced	1/4 cup (35g)
Red onion, chopped	1/4 cup (35g)
Arugula, chopped	1-ounce (25g)
Walnuts, roughly chopped	1 1/2 to 2 tablespoons (10 to 15g)
FOR THE DRESSING	
Extra-virgin olive oil	1 tablespoon
Balsamic vinegar	1 tablespoon
Dash of lemon juice	
FOR A VEGAN OPTION	
Hummus	2 to 3 tablespoons
Cucumber, diced	1/4 cup (35g)
Red onion, chopped	1/4 cup (35g)
1-ounce (25g) arugula, chopped	as you like

Walnuts, roughly chopped	1 1/2 to 2 tablespoons (10 to 15g)

FOR THE VEGAN DRESSING

Extra-virgin olive oil	1 tablespoon
Dash of lemon juice	as you like

SERVES 1

INSTRUCTIONS

1. Entire-wheat pitas are a good way to pile a lot of Sirtfoods in a quick lunch or comfortable and versatile filled meal. You can carry along and get innovative with amounts, but inevitably all you do is stack the additives in and it's nice to go.

Butternut Squash and Date Tagine with Buckwheat

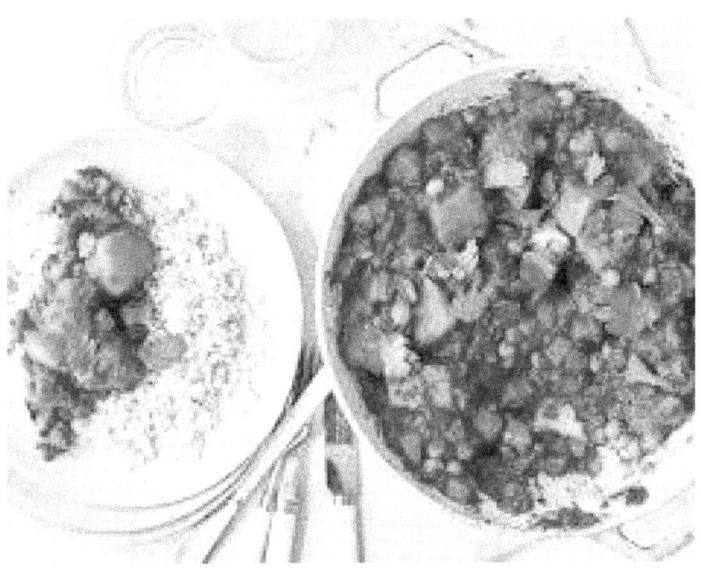

Ingredients	Quantity
Extra virgin olive oil	3 teaspoons
Red onion, finely sliced	1
Finely sliced fresh ginger	1 tablespoon
Garlic cloves, finely sliced	4
Thai chilies, finely sliced	2
Ground cumin	1 tablespoon
Cinnamon stick	1
Ground turmeric	2 tablespoons
Chopped tomatoes	2 x 14-ounce cans (400g each)
Vegetable stock	1 1/4 cups (300ml)
Medjool dates, pitted and chopped	2/3 cup (100g)
of chickpeas, drained and	1 x 14-ounce can (400g)

rinsed	
Butternut squash, peeled and cut into bite-size pieces	2 1/2 cups (500g)
Buckwheat	1 1/4 cups (200g)
Fresh coriander, chopped	2 tablespoons (5g)
Fresh parsley, chopped	1/4 cup (10g)

SERVES 4

INSTRUCTIONS

1. Heat the oven up to 400ºF (200ºC).
2. Cook the oil in 2 teaspoons with the onion, garlic, ginger, and chili for two or three minutes. Insert the cumin and cinnamon and 1 teaspoon of the turmeric, then bake one to two minutes longer.
3. Start adding the tomatoes, stock, dates, and chickpeas and slowly boil for 45-60 minutes. From moment to moment, you may need to insert little more water to accomplish a thick, sticky uniformity and ensure the skillet doesn't run dry.
4. Put the squash in a grilling saucepan, mix with the residual oil and bake till crispy and roasted around the sides for thirty min.
5. Towards the final moment of the cooking process for the tagine, fry the buckwheat with the residual spoonful of turmeric as per the manufacturer guidelines.
6. Start adding the grilled squash and coriander and parsley to the tagine and start serving with buckwheat.

Butter Bean and Miso Dip With Celery Sticks and Oatcakes

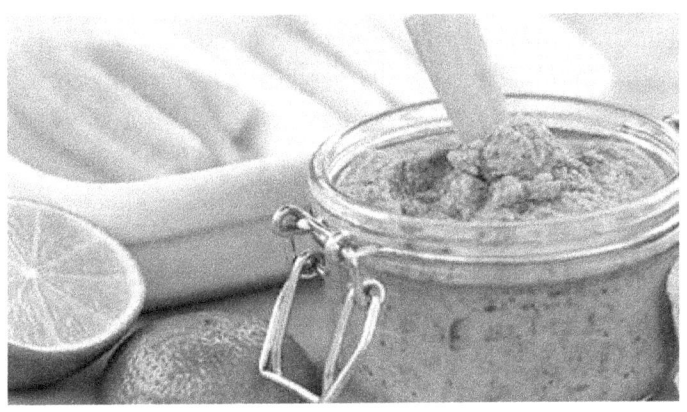

Ingredients	Quantity
Butter beans, drained and rinsed	2 x 14-ounce cans (400g)
Extra virgin olive oil	3 tablespoons
Brown miso paste	2 tablespoons
Juice and grated zest of 1/2 unwaxed lemon	as you like
Medium scallions, trimmed and finely sliced	4
Garlic clove, squeezed	1
Thai chili, finely sliced	1/4
Celery sticks, to serve	as you like
Oatcakes, to serve	as you like

SERVES 4

INSTRUCTIONS

1. Only pound the first 7 components and a potato blender and you'll have a rough combination.
2. Start serving the celery sticks and oatcakes as a sauce.

Yogurt with Berries, Walnuts, and Dark Chocolate

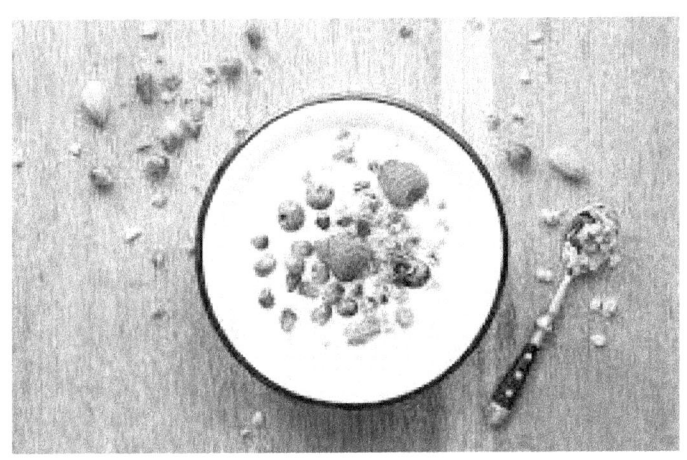

Ingredients	Quantity
Mixed berries	about 1 1/3 cups (125g)
Plain Greek yogurt (or vegan alternative, such as soy or coconut yogurt)	2/3 cup (150g)
Walnuts, chopped	1/4 cup (25g)
Dark chocolate (85 percent cocoa solids), grated	1 1/2 tablespoons (10g)

SERVES 1

INSTRUCTIONS

1. Just add your favorite berries to a pot, and upper surface with the yogurt.
2. Spray with the dark chocolates and the walnuts.

Chicken And Kale Curry With Bombay Potatoes

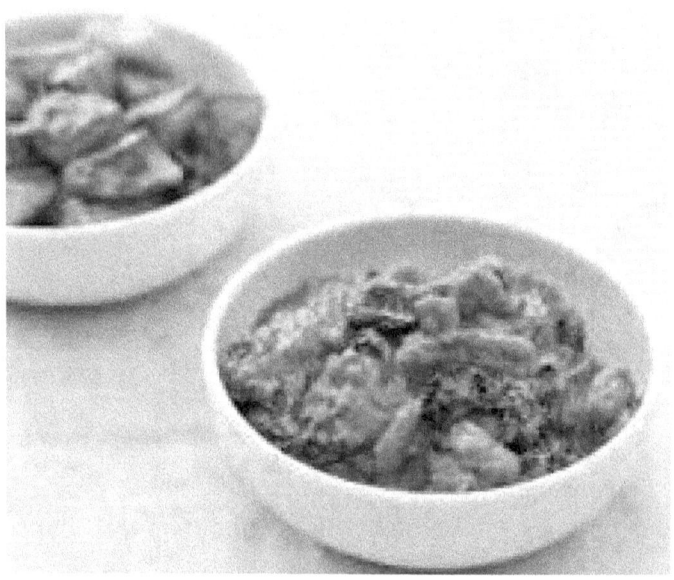

Ingredients	Quantity
Skinless, boneless chicken breasts, cut into bite-size pieces	4 x 4 ½ - to 5 ½ -ounce (120 to 150g)
Extra virgin olive oil	4 tablespoons
Ground turmeric	3 tablespoons
Red onions, sliced	2
Thai chilies, finely sliced	2
Garlic cloves, finely sliced	3
Finely sliced fresh ginger	1 tablespoon
Mild curry powder	1 tablespoon
Can chopped tomatoes	1 x 14-ounce (400g)
Chicken stock	2 $^{1/8}$ cups (500ml)
Coconut milk	7/8 cup (200ml)
Cardamom pods	2

Cinnamon stick	1
Russet potatoes	1 1/3 pounds (600g)
Parsley, chopped	1/4 cup (10g)
Kale, chopped	2 2/3 cups (175g)
Coriander, chopped	2 tablespoons (5g)

SERVES 4

INSTRUCTIONS

1. Massage the chicken breast in one teaspoon of oil, and one tablespoon of turmeric. Mean leaving on for thirty min to marinate.
2. Roast the meat over high temperature (the meat should be fried with adequate oil in the marinade) for four to five minutes just until golden brown all over it and fried fully, after which remove and throw aside.
3. Start heating 1 spoonful of the oil over moderate flame in the roasting pan and insert the onion, chili, garlic and ginger. Roast for about ten minutes till soft, then introduce the curry powder and then another turmeric spoonful and prepare food for more one to two minutes. Append the tomatoes to the pan and allow to roast for another two min. Include the stock, coconut milk, cardamom and cinnamon stick and left for forty-five to sixty minutes to boil. Inspect the pan frequently to make sure it doesn't dry up — you may need to insert more storage.
4. Heat the oven up to 425 ° F (220 ° C). Scrape the potatoes as your gravy is cooking, then slice them into smaller pieces. Put the residual

teaspoon of turmeric in boiling hot water, and simmer for five minutes. Flush well and permit for ten minutes of dry steam. Round every edge they must be white and waxy.
5. Move to a baking dish, mix in the residual oil and grill till nicely browned and crunchy after 30 minutes. When recipe is fully prepared, throw the parsley across.
6. Insert the kale, roasted chicken, and coriander when the sauce has your optimum requirements, and roast for another five minutes to make sure the meat is cooked across, then start serving with the potatoes.

Spiced Scrambled Eggs

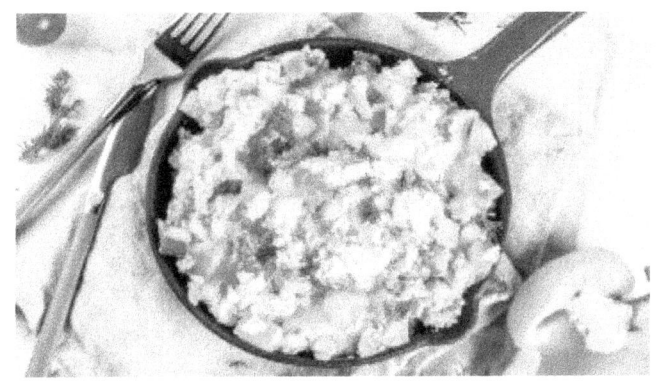

Ingredients	Quantity
Extra virgin olive oil	1 teaspoon
Red onion, finely sliced	1/8 cup (20g)
Thai chili, finely sliced	1/2
Medium eggs	3
Milk	1/4 cup (50ml)
Ground turmeric	1 teaspoon
Parsley, finely sliced	2 tablespoons (5g)

SERVES 1

INSTRUCTIONS

1. In a cooking pot, cook the oil and fried the red onion and chili till smooth but not brown.
2. Blend the eggs, milk, turmeric, and oil next to each other. Insert to the frying skillet and cook for a few minutes over low to moderate heat, starting to move the beaten eggs from around skillet continuously to fumble it and halt it from glued / combustion. Start serving when you have accomplished the uniformity you really want.

Sirt Chili Con Carne

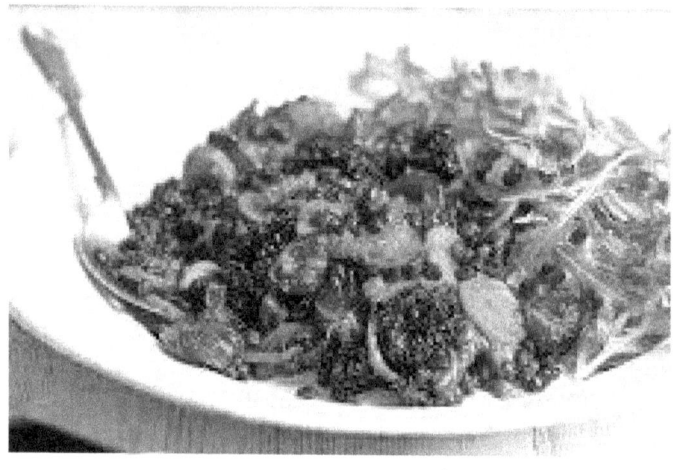

Ingredients	Quantity
Red onion, finely sliced	1
Garlic cloves, finely sliced	3
Thai chilies, finely sliced	2
Extra-virgin olive oil	1 tablespoon
Ground cumin	1 tablespoon
Ground turmeric	1 tablespoon
Lean ground beef (5 percent fat)	1 pound (450g)
Red wine	5/8 cup (150ml)
Red bell pepper, cored, seeds removed and cut into bite-size pieces	1
Cans chopped tomatoes	2 x 14-ounce (400g)
Tomato purée	1 tablespoon

Cocoa powder	1 tablespoon
Canned kidney beans	7/8 cup (150g)
Beef stock	1 1/4 cups (300ml)
Fresh coriander, chopped	2 tablespoons (5g)
Fresh parsley, chopped	2 tablespoons (5g)
Buckwheat	1 cup (160g)

SERVES 4

INSTRUCTIONS

1. Roast the garlic, onion, and chili in the oil for two or three minutes over moderate heat in a large frying pan, then insert the ingredients and continue cooking for a minute or two. Add chopped beef and roast over medium-high temperature for two or three minutes till the meat is well golden brown throughout. Insert the red wine and enable it to steam to reduce by half.
2. Start adding the red pepper, tomatoes, purée tomatoes, cocoa, kidney beans and supply and keep for one hour to boil. Occasionally, you might need to append little more water to accomplish a thick, sticky uniformity. Stir in the sliced spices, right before eating.
3. In the meantime, as per the manufacturer's directions, fry the buckwheat and continue serving alongside the chilli.

Mushroom and Tofu Scramble

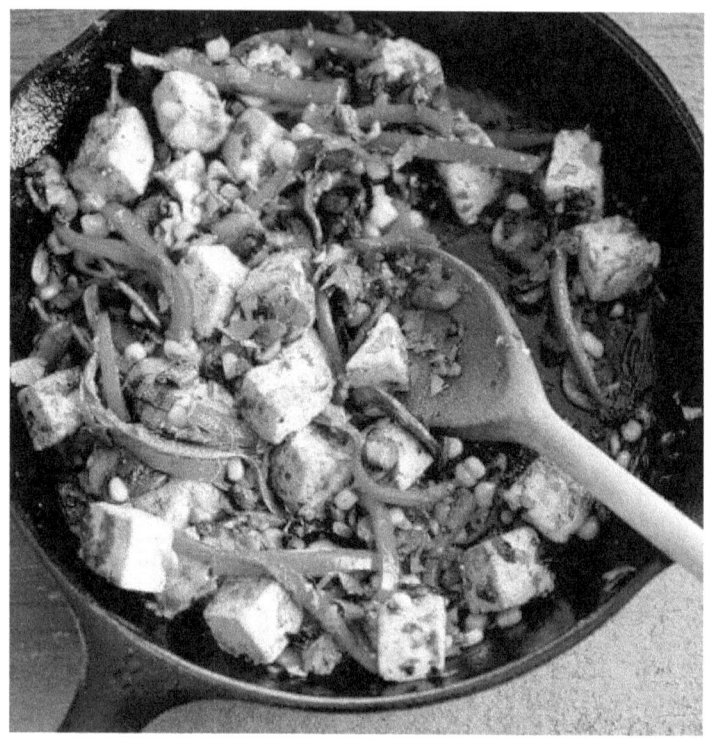

Ingredients	Quantity
Extra-rm tofu	3 1/2 ounces (100g)
Ground turmeric	1 teaspoon
Mild curry powder	1 teaspoon
Kale, roughly chopped	1/3 cup (20g)
Extra virgin olive oil	1 teaspoon
Red onion, thinly sliced	1/8 cup (20g)
Thai chili, thinly sliced	1/2
Mushrooms, thinly sliced	3/4 cup (50g)
Parsley, finely sliced	2 tablespoons (5g)

SERVES 1

INSTRUCTIONS

1. Roll the tofu in cleaned paper and top with anything thick to help drain it.
2. Blend the curry and turmeric powder, then add more water till a light pulp has been accomplished. Heat the Kale for two to three minutes.
3. Warm the oil over medium high heat in a cooking pan and roast the onion, chili, and mushrooms for two or three minutes before browning and softening has begun.
4. Collapse the tofu into bits of small bites and transfer to the saucepan, spill over the tofu the seasoning mixture and completely blend. Fry for two or three minutes over moderate flame so that the ingredients are roasted through and the tofu has begun browning. Add the kale and start cooking for the next minute over moderate flame. Add the parsley, blend well, and serve.

Smoked Salmon Pasta with Chili and Arugula

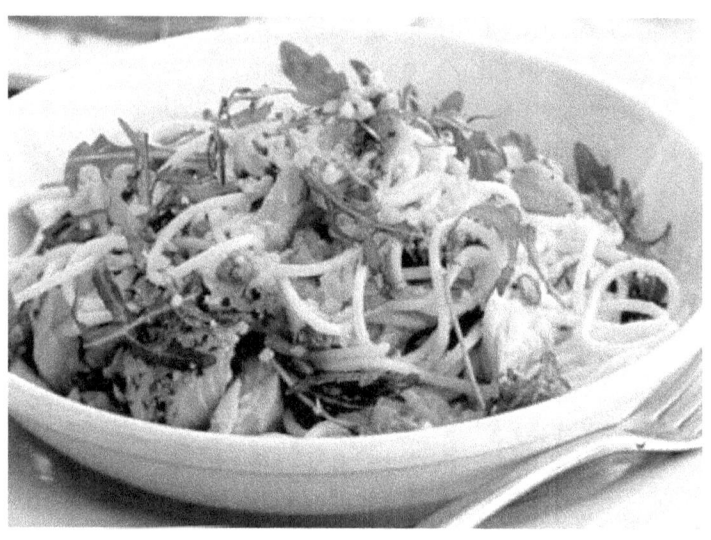

Ingredients	Quantity
Extra virgin olive oil	2 tablespoons
Red onion, finely sliced	1
Garlic cloves, finely sliced	2
Thai chilies, finely sliced	2
Cherry tomatoes, cut in half	1 cup (150g)
White wine	1/2 cup (100ml)
Buckwheat pasta	9 to 11 ounces (250 to 300g)
Smoked salmon	9 ounces (250g)
Capers	2 tablespoons
Juice of lemon	½
Arugula	2 ounces (60g)
Parsley, chopped	1/4 cup (10g)

SERVES 4

INSTRUCTIONS

1. In a broiler pan start cooking one teaspoon of the oil over moderate flame. Stir in the onion, garlic, chili, and fry till smooth but not dark brown.
2. Start adding the tomatoes and permit to bake for one or two minutes. To minimize by half, append the white wine and bubble.
3. Bake the pasta in hot water with one tablespoon of oil for eight to ten minutes based on whether you like it to serve, then rinse.
4. Split the salmon into pieces and apply the capers, lemon juice, arugula, parsley, and the tomato into saucepan. Insert the sauce, blend together, and eat straight away. Sprinkle some oil over top.

Buckwheat Pasta Salad

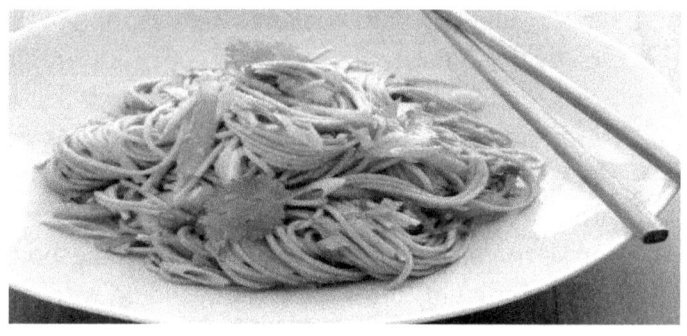

Ingredients	Quantity
Buckwheat pasta, cooked according to the package instructions	2 ounces (50g)
Handful of arugulas	large
Handful of basil leaves	small
Cherry tomatoes, cut in half	8
Avocado, diced	1/2
Olives	10
Extra-virgin olive oil	1 tablespoon
Pine nuts	2 1/2 tablespoons (20g)

SERVES 1

INSTRUCTIONS

Incorporate all the spices, except for the pine nuts, delicately and organize them on a tray, then disperse the nuts over its top.

Buckwheat Pancakes with Strawberries, Dark Chocolate Sauce, and Squeezed Walnuts

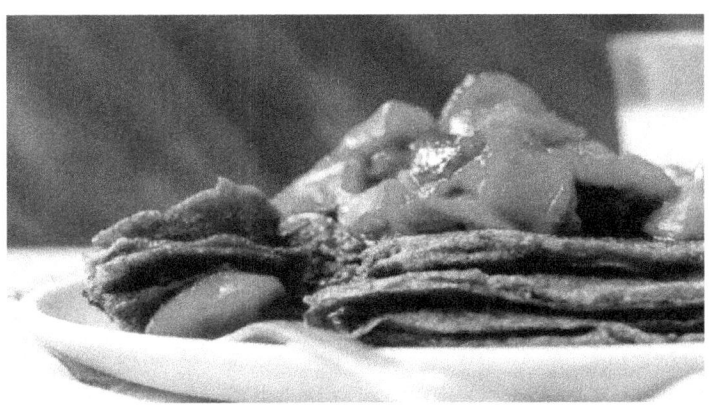

Ingredients	Quantity
FOR THE PANCAKES	
Milk	1 1/2 cups (350ml)
Buckwheat our	7/8 cup (150g)
Large egg	1
Extra-virgin olive oil, for cooking	1 tablespoon
FOR THE CHOCOLATE SAUCE	
Dark chocolate (85 percent cocoa solids)	3 1/2 ounces (100g)
Milk	1/3 cup (85ml)
Double cream	1 tablespoon
Extra-virgin olive oil	1 tablespoon
TO SERVE	
Strawberries, hulled and chopped	2 cups (400g)
Walnuts, chopped	7/8 cup (100g)

MAKES 6 TO 8 PANCAKES, DEPENDING ON THE SIZE

INSTRUCTIONS

1. Add all ingredients besides the olive oil in a food processor to start making the pancake sauce and mix till you have a smooth blend. It must not be too dense or too runny. (Any leftover mixture can be kept in an enclosed jar or in your refrigerator for up to five days. Make sure to blend properly before using it again.)
2. Melt the dark chocolate in a warmth-proof bowl over a tray of boiling water to produce the chocolate sauce. When warmed, blend well in the milk, and whisk vigorously, then append the double cream and olive oil. By keeping the water in the oven, you can maintain the sauce hot, boiling at very low flame till your pancakes are prepared.
3. Microwave a small and medium heavy lower part frying pan till it begins smoking, then append the olive oil to begin making the pancakes.
4. Place some of the mixture into the middle of the bowl, then move the excess mixture around it till you've coated the entire surface; you might need to apply a little more mixture to do that. If your saucepan is hot sufficient, you would just need to bake the pancake from each side for one minute or so.
5. Using a spatula to remove the pancake around the bottom, until you can see it go dark around the top, then turn this over. Attempt to turn over

and prevent splitting it in one move. But at the other side, fry for another moment or so, and move to a tray.
6. Put some strawberries in the middle and slide the pancake upwards. Proceed till you've made many more pancakes, as necessary.
7. Across each pancake, scoop a decent amount of marinade and scatter with certain sliced walnuts.
8. You will notice your initial attempts to be much too fatty or to fell apart, but if you reach the formula for your mixture that fits better for you and you refine your method, you'll make it like an expert. For this scenario makes preparation good.

Tofu and Shiitake Mushroom Soup

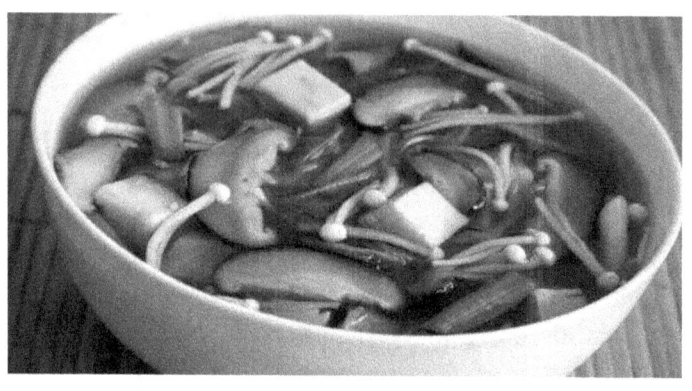

Ingredients	Quantity
Dried wakame (seaweed)	1/3 ounce (10g)
Vegetable stock	1-quart (1 liter)
Shiitake mushrooms, sliced	7 ounces (200g)
Miso paste	1/3 cup (120g)
Block rm tofu, cut into small cubes	1 x 14-ounce (400g)
Scallions, trimmed and sliced on the diagonal	2
Thai chili, finely sliced (optional)	1

SERVES 4

INSTRUCTIONS

1. Drench the wakame for ten minutes in hot water then rinse. Introduce the stock to a simmer, then introduce the mushrooms and delicately boil for 1-2 minutes.
2. Dissociate the miso paste with a few of the hot stocks in a pan to guarantee it completely be dissolved. Apply the miso and tofu to the remaining inventory, be careful to not let the soup simmer because that will ruin the delicate taste of miso. When using and serving, add the soaked wakame, scallions, and chili.

Sirtfood Bites

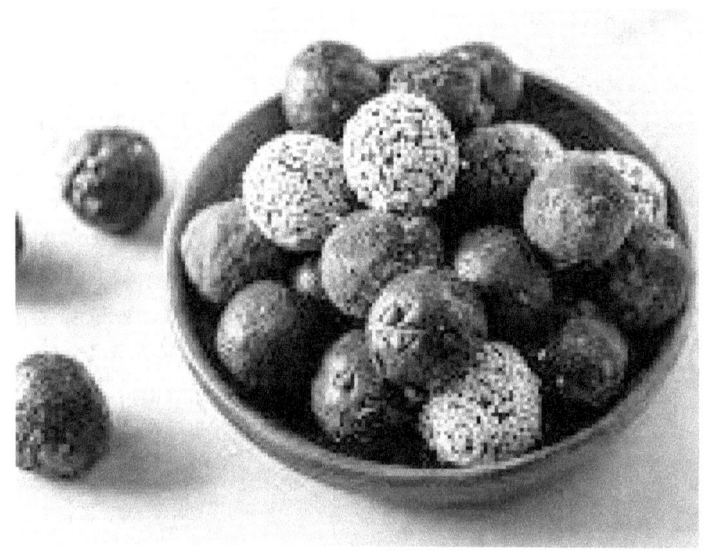

Ingredients	Quantity
Walnuts	1 cup (120g)
Dark chocolate (85 percent cocoa solids), broken into pieces; or 1/4 cup Cocoa nibs	1 ounce (30g)
Medjool dates, pitted	9 ounces (250g)
Cocoa powder	1 tablespoon
Ground turmeric	1 tablespoon
Extra-virgin olive oil	1 tablespoon
The scraped seeds OR vanilla extract	1 vanilla pod OR 1 teaspoon
Water	1 to 2 tablespoons

MAKES 15 TO 20 BITES

INSTRUCTIONS

1. Put the walnuts and dark chocolate in a food processor and pulse them till the powder is perfect.
2. Append all the rest of the ingredients apart from water and blend until the solution turned into a ball. Ensure the reliability and validity of the paste, you might not have to apply the water-you mayn't want it to be so messy.
3. Make the combination into bite-size pellets using your palms and cool in an enclosed jar for at least one hour until eating them. With any more chocolate or dry coconut, you might roll any of the pullet to make a separate texture, if you prefer. They should store it in your refrigerator for up to one week.

Quinoa, Chickpea and Turmeric Curry

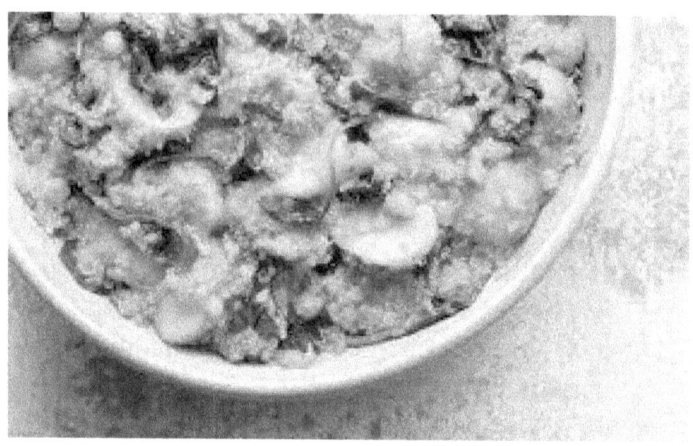

Ingredients	Quantity
New potatoes, cut in half	500g
Garlic cloves, squeeze	3
Ground turmeric	3 teaspoons
Ground coriander	1 teaspoon
Chilli flakes or (powder)	1 teaspoon
Ground ginger	1 teaspoon
Chopped tomatoes	400g
Coconut milk	400g
Tomato purée	1 tablespoon
Pepper and salt	as you like
Quinoa	180g
Chickpeas, drained and rinsed	400g
Spinach	150g

Serves 6

INSTRUCTIONS

1. Put the potatoes in a bowl with cool water and bring them to the flame, then let them steam for around 25 minutes before a knife is comfortably sticked across. Flush them good.
2. In a large saucepan, put the potatoes and add the garlic, turmeric, coriander, chili, ginger, coconut milk, tomato purée and tomatoes. Bring to a simmer, season with pepper and salt, then put a mug from just boiled 300ml water into the quinoa.
3. Significantly decrease heat to a simmer, put on the cover and encourage cooking. Mix every five minutes, or so, within the next thirty minutes to ensure that nothing tends to stick to the lower part. (This is such a long time to prepare, but that is how long it would take to prepare quinoa in all these additives, not only in water.) Midway through frying, add the chickpeas. When just five minutes are remaining, insert the spinach and whisk it into before it wilts. Once the quinoa has baked and is fluffy, it's prepared, not crunchy.

If you want a touch of fire, apply a sliced red chili at the very same time as all the other peppers to the frying curry.

Savory Turmeric Pancakes with Lemon Yogurt Sauce

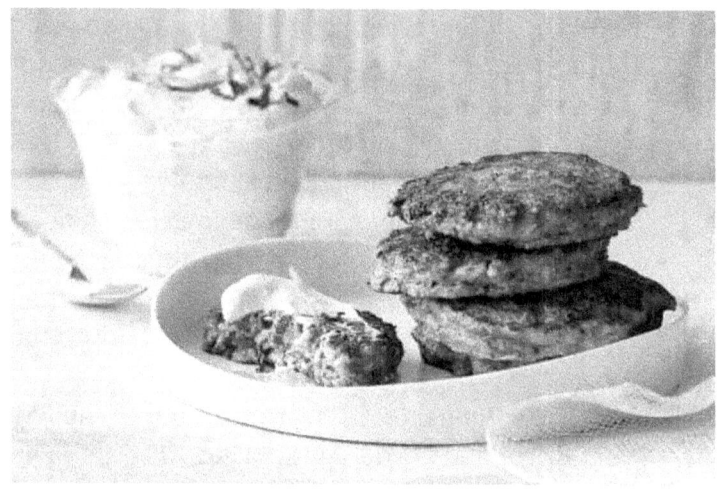

For The Pancakes

Ingredients	Quantity
Ground turmeric	2 teaspoons
Ground cumin	1½ teaspoons
Salt	1 teaspoon
Ground coriander	1 teaspoon
Garlic powder	½ teaspoon
Ground black pepper	½ teaspoon freshly
Head broccoli, cut into florets	1
Large eggs, lightly beaten	3
Plain unsweetened almond milk	2 tablespoons

Almond flour	1 cup
Coconut oil	4 teaspoons

Serves 8 pancakes

For The Yogurt Sauce

Ingredients	**Quantity**
Greek yogurt	1 cup plain
Garlic clove, minced	1
Lemon juice (from 1 lemon), to taste	1 to 2 tablespoons
Ground turmeric	¼ teaspoon
Mint leaves (fresh), minced	10
Lemon zest (from 1 lemon)	2 teaspoons

INSTRUCTIONS

1. Make the sauce to yogurt. In a cup, add the yoghurt, garlic, lemon juice, turmeric, mint, and zest. Where appropriate, try and spice with more citrus juice. Set aside or put it in the fridge until prepare for eating.
2. Make pancakes. Blend the turmeric, cumin, salt, coriander, garlic, and pepper into a shallow pot.
3. Put the broccoli in a blender. blend into tiny chunks until the florets are shattered. Move the broccoli to a large mixing bowl, then put the eggs, almond milk, and almond flour. Remove the spice mixture, and merge well.
4. Heat 1 teaspoon of the coconut oil over medium to low temperature in a non - stick frying pan. Pour 1/4 batter into your pan. Heat the pancake until there are tiny rises on the top, and the base

is light brown, 2 to 3 minutes. Switch over and bake the pancake for another 2 to 3 minutes. Transmit the baked pancakes to an oven-safe dish and put them in a 200 ° F oven to retain them warm.
5. Keep making the 3 pancakes left, use the residual oil and batter.

Blueberry Smoothie

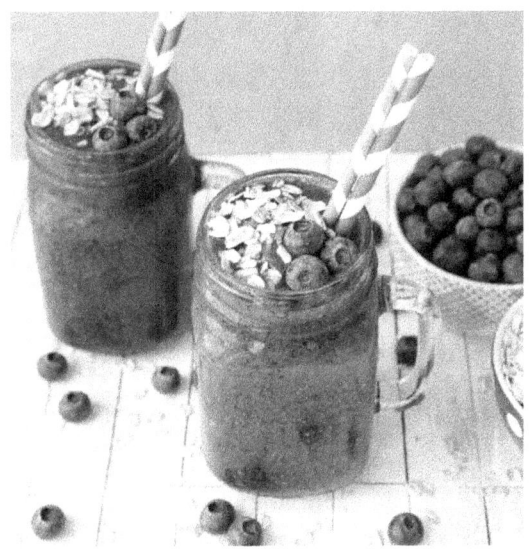

Ingredients	Quantity
Ripe banana	1
Blueberries	100g
Blackberries	100g
Natural yogurt	2 tablespoons
Milk	200ml
Calories	160
Ready in	2 minutes

Serves 2

INSTRUCTIONS

This yogurt smoothie has a rich, creamy taste.

1. Mix together all of the food items until all become light and fluffy.

Blueberry Banana Pancakes with Chunky Apple Compote and Golden Turmeric Latte

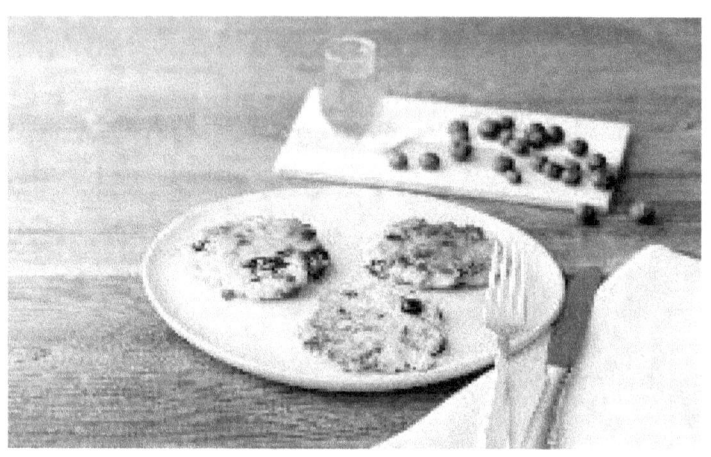

Blueberry Banana Pancakes

Ingredients	Quantity
Bananas	6
Eggs	6
Rolled oats	150g
Baking powder	2 teaspoons
Salt	¼ teaspoon
Blueberries	25g

Chunky Apple Compote

Ingredients	Quantity
Apples	2
dates (pitted)	5
lemon juice	1 tablespoon
cinnamon powder	1/4 teaspoon
pinch salt	as you like

Golden Turmeric Latte

Ingredients	Quantity

Coconut milk	3 cups
Turmeric powder	1 teaspoon
Cinnamon powder	1 teaspoon
Raw honey	1 teaspoon
Black pepper (increases absorption)	Pinch
Ginger root (fresh and peeled)	Tiny piece
Cayenne pepper (optional)	Pinch

INSTRUCTIONS

For the Blueberry Banana Pancakes

1. In a high-speed blender, put the rolled oats and process for 1 minute or until an oat flour has developed. Bit of advice: please ensure your processor is really dry before you do this or else it's all going to get damp!
2. Now introduce the bananas, eggs, baking powder and salt to the mixer and pulse to form a smooth batter for two min.
3. Carefully transfer and fold in the blueberries to a large mixing bowl. Allow the baking powder to sit for 10 minutes until it triggers.
4. To make your pancakes, introduce a dollop of butter to your cooking pans over medium-high fire (this will make them very fluffy and crispy!). Insert some spoons of the blueberry pancake mix and fry on the downstream part for until perfectly golden. Put the pancake into the other side to cook.

For the Chunky Apple Compote

1. Chop the apples to the center and rough.
2. Place all in a food processor with 2 spoonsful of water and a sprinkle of salt. Pulse your chunky apple compote to shape.

For the Golden Turmeric Latte

1. In a high-speed mixer, combine all ingredients unless these become smooth.
2. Spill over moderate flame into a small saucepan and cook for 4 minutes until heated but not boiling.
3. Enjoy!

Buckwheat Superfood Muesli

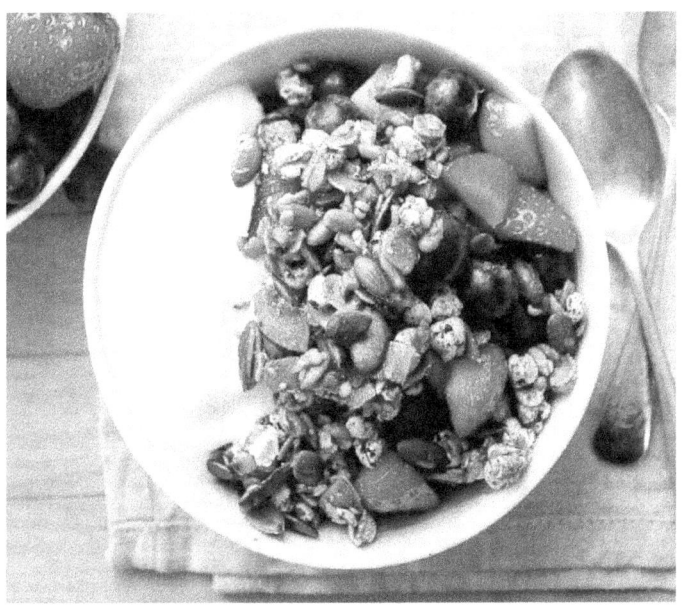

Ingredients	Quantity
Buckwheat flukes	20g
Buckwheat puffs	10g
Desiccated coconut or coconut flakes	15g
Medjool dates (pitted and chopped)	40g
Walnuts, finely sliced	15g
Cocoa nibs	10g
Strawberries (chopped and hulled)	100g
Plain Greek yogurt OR vegan alternative like (soy or coconut yogurt)	100g

INSTRUCTIONS

Mix all the above-mentioned components together (end up leaving out the strawberries and yogurt if not eaten immediately).

NOTES

Just mix the remaining ingredients and place them in an airtight jar if you'd like to make this in stock or cook it the night ahead. The very next day all you have to do is insert the strawberries and yogurt and it's nice to go.

Mocha Chocolate Mousse

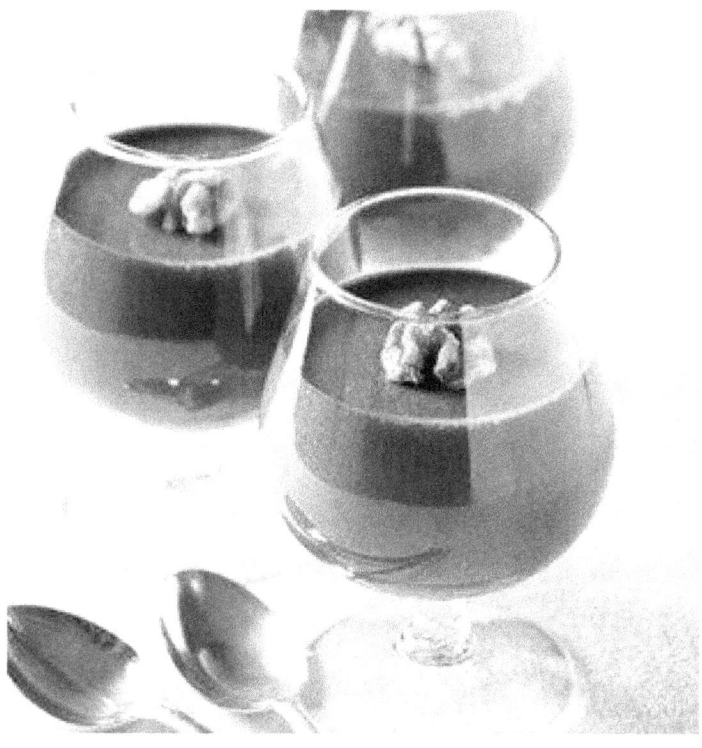

Everybody appreciates mousse in chocolate and this one has a beautiful beam and airy shape. It's fast and easy to make, and usually best served the day after it's done.

Ingredients	Quantity
Dark chocolate (cocoa solids 85%)	250g
Medium free-range eggs (separated)	6
Strong black coffee	4 tablespoons
Almond milk	4 tablespoons
Chocolate coffee beans	to decorate

Serves 4–6

INSTRUCTIONS

1. Melt the chocolate in a bowl of softly bubbling water in a large tub, ensuring the tub 's lower surface doesn't contact the surface. Turn off the heat and remove the bowl and allow the molten chocolate to cool at room temperature.
2. When the melting chocolate has achieved ambient temperature, swirl one at a time in the egg yolks and then add softly in the coffee and almond milk.
3. Stir the egg whites with a manual electric mixer until sharp peaks form, then add a few heaping spoonsful into the chocolate mixture to soften it. Roll in the remainder softly, use a big steel spoon.
4. Move the mousse to single glasses and smooth the color. Protect for at least 2 hours, preferably overnight, with a plastic wrap and chill. Until eating, adorn with chocolate coffee beans.

Raw Brownie Bites

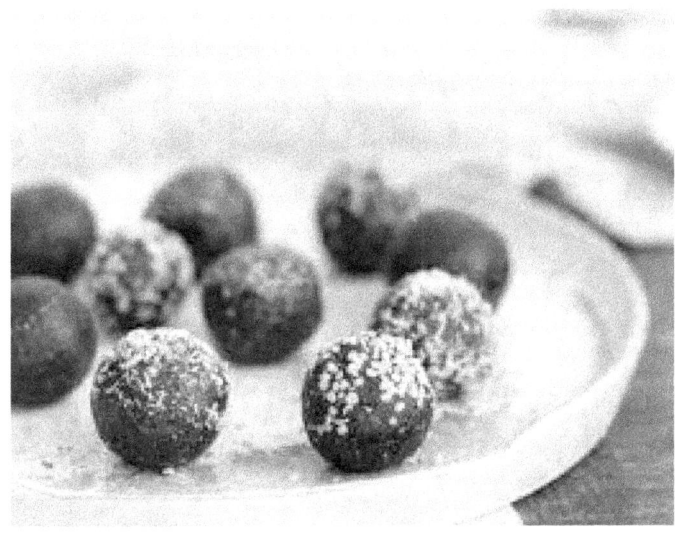

Ingredients	Quantity
Whole walnuts	2½ cups
Almonds	¼ cup
Medjool dates	2½ cups
Cacao powder	1 cup
Vanilla extract	1 teaspoon
Sea salt	⅛ - ¼ teaspoon
Total Time	**5 minutes**

Serves 6

INSTRUCTIONS

1. Put everything in a mixing bowl till it is well put together.
2. Put on a cookie sheet and roll into rollers and refrigerate for thirty min or chill in the fridge for two hours.

Moroccan Spiced Eggs

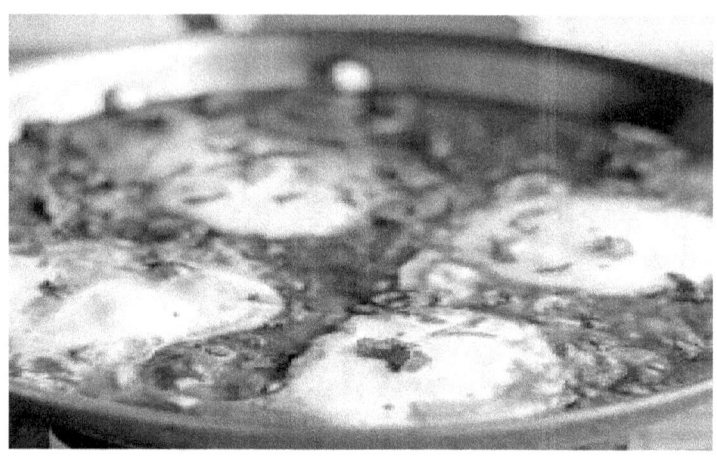

Ingredients	Quantity
Olive oil	1 teaspoon
Shallot (finely sliced and peeled)	1
Red (bell) pepper, (deseeded and finely sliced)	1
Garlic clove, (peeled and finely sliced)	1
Courgette (zucchini), (peeled and finely sliced)	1
Tomato puree (paste)	1 tablespoon
Mild chili powder	½ teaspoon
Ground cinnamon	¼ teaspoon
Ground cumin	¼ teaspoon
Salt	½ teaspoon
Chopped tomatoes	1 × 400g (14oz)
Chickpeas in water	1 × 400g (14oz)
Flat-leaf parsley (small handful)	10g (1/3oz)

Medium eggs	4 at room temperature
Calories	**394**
READY IN	**50 MINUTES**

Serves 2

INSTRUCTIONS

1. In a frying pan, heat the oil, insert the shallot and red (bell) pepper and cook softly for five min. Stir in the garlic and courgette (zucchini) and cook for a few minutes. Insert the tomato puree (paste), salt and spices and mix in.
2. Apply the sliced tomatoes and chickpeas (soaking liquor and all) to a moderate fire. Boil the sauce for thirty min with the cover off the pan – please ensure, it bubbles softly throughout, and encourage it to decrease by around one-third in capacity.
3. Lift the sliced parsley from the fire and stir throughout.
4. Set the microwave temperature to 200C/180C fan/350F.
5. Take the tomato sauce to a moderate boiling when you are ready to cook the eggs, and switch to a clean, oven-proof bowl.
6. Smash the eggs to the edge of the platter and slowly drop them into the stew. Wrap in foil, then bake for 10-15 minutes of cooking. Start serving the concoction with the eggs remaining atop in small cups.

Vietnamese Turmeric Fish with Herbs & Mango Sauce

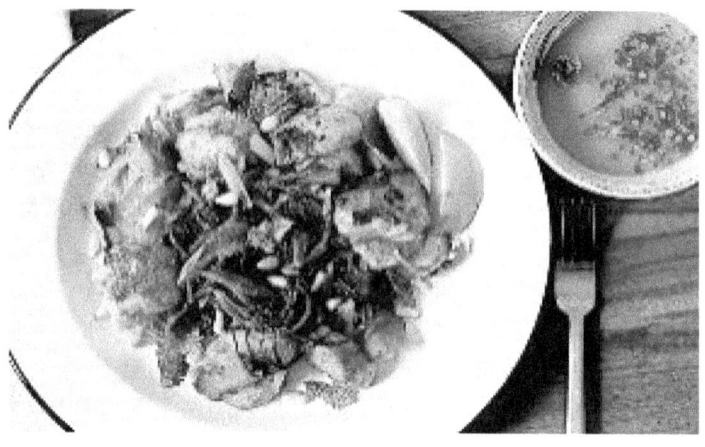

Fish

Ingredients	Quantity
Fresh cod fish (skinless and boneless), cut it ½ inch thick and about 2-inch piece wide	1 ¼ lbs.
Coconut oil in pan and fry the fish	2 tablespoons (plus a few more tablespoon if necessary)
Sea salt to taste	Small pinch of

Fish marinade

Ingredients	Quantity
Turmeric powder	1 tablespoon
Sea salt	1 teaspoon
Chinese cooking wine OR dry	1 tablespoon

sherry	
Minced ginger	2 teaspoons
Olive oil	2 tablespoons

Marinate for at least 1 hr.

Infused Scallion and Dill Oil

Ingredients	Quantity
Scallions (slice into long thin shape)	2 cups
Fresh dill	2 cups of
Sea salt to taste	Pinch

Mango dipping sauce

Ingredients	Quantity
Medium sized ripe mango	1
Rice vinegar	2 tablespoons
Juice of lime	½
Garlic clove	1
Dry red chili pepper (stir in before serving)	1 teaspoon

Toppings

Fresh cilantro	as you like
Lime juice	as you like
Nuts (pine nuts or cashew)	as you like

Prep time: 15 mins Cook time 30 mins Total 45 minutes

Serves: 4

INSTRUCTIONS

1. Marinate the fish for one hour or as long as it is overnight.
2. Add all ingredients in a mixing bowl under "Mango Dipping Sauce," and combine until quality is obtained.

To Pan-Fry The Fish:

1. Heat 2 tablespoons of coconut oil over high temperature in a big, nonstick skillet. Add the premarinated fish if hot. Note: put the fish slices separately in the saucepan and segregate them into two or more quantities for frying if needed.
2. A loud sizzle should be heard, upon which you can reduce the heat to moderate heat.
3. Do not turn or relocate the fish till after, about 5 minutes, you see a golden-brown skin tone on the side. Top with a tablespoon of sea salt. If required add more coconut oil to cook the fish.
4. When the fish is in golden brown, move the fish gently on the other side on cook. Transmit onto a large plate once it's accomplished. Note: The saucepan should have some residual oil in it. We use the remaining oil to make oil that is infused with scallion and dill.

To Make The Scallion And Dill Infused Oil:

1. Just use rest of the oil over medium to high heat in the frying pan, add 2 cups of scallions and 2

cups of dill. Remove from the heat once the scallions and dill are introduced. Start giving them a delicate flip, about fifteen seconds, till the scallions and dill simmered. Season with a sprinkle of salt at sea.
2. Plop the scallion, dill and infused oil over the fish and represent fresh cilantro, lime, and nuts with mango sauce.

Sirtfood Diet's Shakshuka

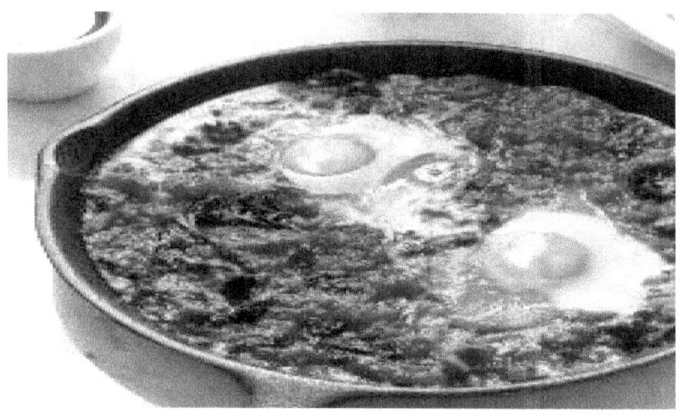

Ingredients	Quantity
Extra virgin olive oil	1 teaspoon
Red onion, finely sliced	40g
Garlic clove, finely sliced	1
Celery, finely sliced	30g
Bird's eye chili, finely sliced	1
Ground cumin	1 teaspoon
Ground turmeric	1 teaspoon
Paprika	1 teaspoon
Tinned chopped tomatoes	400g
Kale, stems removed, finely sliced	30g
Chopped parsley	1 tablespoon
Medium eggs	2
Preparation time	**40 minutes**

Serves 1

INSTRUCTIONS

1. Cook over medium – low heat a small, depth-sided saucepan. Add the oil and brown the onion, garlic, celery, chili, and spices for approximately one minute.
2. Remove the tomatoes, and leave the sauce to boil slowly, stirring regularly for twenty minutes.
3. Add the kale and continue cooking for another five minutes. When you thought the sauce is too stiff, just apply a bit of water. Mix in the parsley if your sauce has a good rich flavor.
4. Made in the sauce two tiny wells, then break each egg onto them. Lower the heat to its lowest level and use a seal or foil to protect the oven. Left the eggs for ten to twelve minutes to cook, where the whites will be firm while the yolks are still sticky. Reheat for an extra three to four minutes if you like strong yolks. Serve right away- preferably directly from the pan.

Sirtfood Diet's Braised Puy Lentils

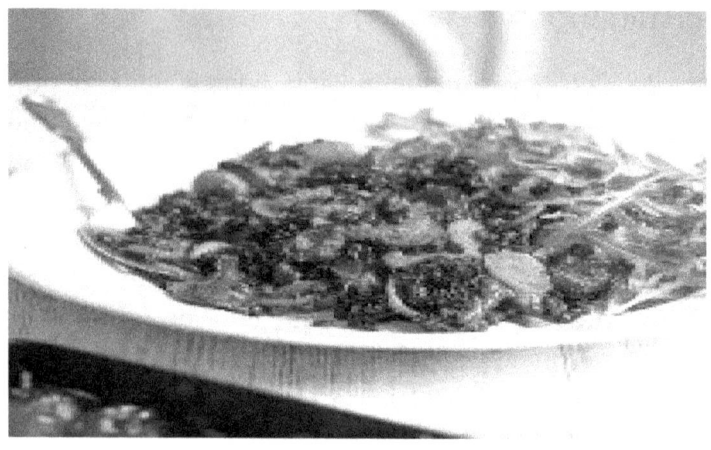

Ingredients	Quantity
Cherry tomatoes, cut in half	8
Extra virgin olive oil	2 teaspoons
Red onion (thinly sliced)	40 g
Garlic clove, finely sliced	1
Celery (thinly sliced)	40 g
Carrots (thinly sliced and peeled)	40 g
Paprika	1 teaspoon
Thyme (fresh or dry)	1 teaspoon
Puy lentils	75 g
Vegetable stock	220 ml
Kale, finely sliced	50 g
Parsley, finely sliced	1 tablespoon
Rocket	20 g
Preparation time	40 – 50 minutes

Serves: 1

INSTRUCTIONS

1. Heat the oven up to 120ºC/gas ½.
2. Place the tomatoes in a small roasting tin and fry for thirty-five to forty minutes in the oven.
3. Cook a casserole over low – moderate heat. Add a tablespoon of olive oil with red onion, garlic, celery, and carrot and cook till loosened for one to two minutes. Stir in the thyme then paprika, then simmer for another minute.
4. Wash the lentils in a really well-meshed sieve and insert them together with the stock to the saucepan. Bring to a simmer, then rising heat and slowly boil with a cover on the pot for twenty minutes. Start giving the pan a swirl after about seven minutes, providing some water if the level is too much low.
5. Stir in the kale and prepare food for another ten minutes. Mix in the parsley and roasted tomatoes when the lentils are baked. Represent the residual teaspoon of olive oil with a rocket sprinkled.

Salmon Sirt Super Salad

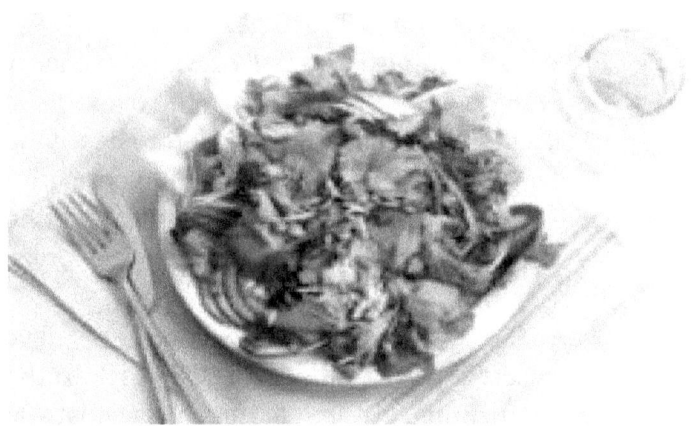

Ingredients	Quantity
Rocket	50g
Chicory leaves	50g
Smoked salmon slices (alt. cooked chicken breast, lentils, or tinned tuna)	100g
Avocado (stoned, sliced and peeled)	80g
Celery (sliced)	40g
Red onion (sliced)	20g
Walnuts, finely sliced	15g
Capers	1 tbs
Large Medjool date (chopped and pitted)	1
Extra-virgin olive oil	1 tbs
Juice of lemon	¼
Parsley, finely sliced	10g
Celery leaves or lovage, finely sliced	10g

INSTRUCTIONS

1. Organize the leaves of the salad over a serving dish. Blend all the rest of the ingredients and represent over the leaves.

Chinese-Style Pork with Pak Choi

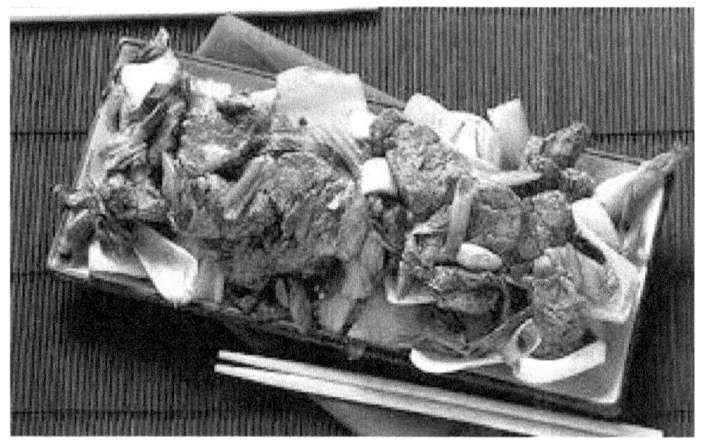

Ingredients	Quantity
Firm tofu (cut into large cubes)	400g
Corn flour	1 tablespoon
Water	1 tablespoon
Chicken stock	125ml
Rice wine	1 tablespoon
Tomato puree	1 tablespoon
Brown sugar	1 teaspoon
Soy sauce	1 tablespoon
Clove garlic (squeezed and peeled)	1
Fresh ginger (grated and peeled)	1 thumb (5cm)
Rapeseed oil	1 tablespoon
Shiitake mushrooms (sliced)	100g
Shallot (sliced and peeled)	1
Choi sum or pak choi (cut into thin Slices, pork mince)	200g, 400g (10% fat)

Beansprouts	100g
Large handful parsley, finely sliced	(20g)
CALORIES	**377**

Serves: 4

INSTRUCTIONS

1. Put the tofu out on paper for the fridge, fill with far more paper for the fridge and put aside.
2. Blend the corn flour and water in a tiny bowl, attempting to remove all the lumps. Stir in the stock of poultry, rice wine, tomato puree, brown sugar, and soy sauce. Insert the squeezed garlic and ginger, then stir.
3. Heat the oil to an elevated temperature in a wok, or large deep fryer. Attach the shiitake mushrooms, and stir-fry until fried and glossy for two to three minutes. Start by removing the mushrooms from the skillet and set aside with a slotted spoon. Insert the tofu to the saucepan and stir-fry all sides until golden. Cover with a knife, then cast aside.
4. Add the shallot and choi pak to the wok, stir-fry for two minutes, then add the mince. Fry until the slim is heated through, then insert the sauce, decrease a notch of heat, and enable the sauce to steam for a couple of minutes around the meat. Attach the beansprouts, mushrooms shiitake and tofu to the saucepan and cook up. Turn off heat, mix in the parsley and instantly start serving.

Chapter 7
How to Lose Fat

List of Sirtuin activating, fat burning SIRTfoods

SIRTfoods contain naturally occurring compounds that are known to activate sirtuin proteins. These sirtuin activators include powerful antioxidants called polyphenols.

Almond	Apple cider vinegar	Apples
Apricots	Asparagus	Aubergine/eggplant
Avocado	Balsamic vinegar	Bananas
Bean sprouts	Bell peppers	Blackcurrants
Black garlic	Black grapes	Blueberries
Brazil nuts	Broccoli	Buckwheat
Cabbages	Capers	Carrot
Cauliflower	Celeriac	Celery
Cherries	Chia seeds	Chickpeas (garbanzo beans)

Chicory	Chillies	Cocoa
Coconut	Coffee	Corn
Cranberries	Dark chocolate	Dates
Eggs	Elderberries	Fava (broad) beans
Fennel	Figs	Flaxseed
Garlic	Globe artichokes	Goji berries
Gooseberries	Grapefruit	Guava
Hazelnuts	Horseradish	Kale
Kidney beans	Lemons	Lentils
Lettuce	Limes	Macadamia nuts
Mango	Mangosteen	Miso soup
Mushrooms	Oily fish	Olives
Olive oil	Onions	Oranges
Pak choi / bok choy	Papaya	Passion fruit
Peanuts	Pears	Pecans
Physalis (Cape gooseberry)	Pine nuts	Pineapple
Pistachios	Plums	Pomegranate
Prunes	Pumpkin	Pumpkin seeds
Purple Potato	Red Grapes	Red kidney beans
Red onions	Rocket (arugula)	Rye
Soybeans	Spinach	Strawberries
Sweetcorn	Sweet potato	Tomatoes
Walnuts	Watercress	Watermelon

Herbs and spices

Most of the herbs and the spices are powerful sirtuin activators, including clove, black pepper, cinnamon, cardamom, cumin, coriander, lemon verbena, mint, ginger, oregano, nutmeg, rosemary, parsley, thyme, sage, turmeric, and edible flowers.

Fat burning drinks

Green tea, Black tea, White tea, Matcha, Chamomile tea, Rooibos and Red wine (one glass per day).

If you ate nothing but the above foods, you would definitely lose weight!

Chapter 8
Maintain a healthy life

Doing exercise with the diet

The Sirtfood Diet is about eating those foods that are designed to promote sustained weight loss and well-being by nature. Even with the advantages that you see from adopting the diet, you might slip into the pit of feeling there's no need to exercise. This will be endorsed by many diet books, saying how ineffective exercise is compared with following the right diet for weight loss. And it is right; we can't exercise bad diet. It's not the way we saw earlier that was intended to drive weight loss. It is expensive, and there are too many frontiers to be negative.

So, it's true that till we see stars or perform an Olympian's feats there's no need to pound the treadmill — but what about general everyday movement?

The truth is we are now much less involved than we used to be. The age of technology has ensured that physical activity is practically factored out of our everyday lives with all the changes it has provided. We don't really have to bother with the whole business of being active, unless we actually want to. We can roll out of bed, drive to work, take the elevator, sit at a desk the whole day, drive home, eat and watch TV before rolling back into bed, then do the same the next day and the next day.

Whatever sport or physical activity you enjoy is appropriate. Pleasure and exercise do not have to be mutually exclusive! And their social aspect enriches team or community sports even more. It's also about everyday things like taking the bike instead of the car, or getting off the bus one stop earlier, or just parking farther away to increase the distance you've got to walk around. Take the stairs and not the elevator. Go outside and garden with do some. Play in the park with your family or get more out with the dog. Everything counts. Anything that has you up and going will activate your sirtuin genes frequently and at moderate strength, maximizing the benefits of the Sirtfood Diet.

Engaging in physical activity while eating a diet rich in Sirtfood gives your buck the maximum sirtuin bang.

Sirtfood diet during pregnancy

The Sirtfood Diet isn't recommended if you're trying to conceive, or if you're pregnant or nursing. It is a powerful diet for weight loss which makes it inappropriate. Don't put off eating plenty of Sirtfoods though, as these are exceptionally healthy foods to be included as part of a balanced and varied pregnancy diet.

The truth is we are now much less involved than we used to be. The age of technology has ensured that physical activity is practically factored out of our everyday lives with all the changes it has provided. We don't really have to bother with the whole business of being active, unless we actually want to.

Sirtfood diet for children

Sirtfood diet is not intended for children. This doesn't mean children will miss out on the excellent health benefits that are provided by having more Sirtfoods in their overall diet. A large majority of Sirt foods are extremely healthy foods for children or help them attain balanced or nutritious diets. Many of the recipes planned for the stage 2 diet were produced with families in mind including the children's taste buds. The likes of the Sirtfood pizza, the chili con carne and the Sirtfood bites are perfect child-friendly foods with a higher nutritional value than usual food offerings for children.

Although most Sirtfoods are extremely healthy for children to eat, the green juice, which is too concentrated in fat burning sirtfoods, is not recommended. We also advise against important caffeine sources, such as coffee and green tea.

Sirtfood diet for people on medication

The Sirtfood Diet is perfect to many people, but it can alter the processes of certain diseases and the drug acts recommended by your doctor due to its powerful effects on fat burning and wellbeing. Similarly, other medications are not ideal in a fasting condition.

During the Sirtfood Diet trial, each individual's suitability was assessed before they embarked on the diet, particularly those taking medication. Obviously, we can't do that for you, so if you're suffering from a major health problem, taking prescribed medicines, or have other reasons to worry about getting on a diet.

Cancer Prevention Foods

All cancer and nutrition studies point to eating plant-based foods for their phytonutrients and other special compounds. Target for five to nine regular fruit and vegetables of all kinds — especially these six megastars.

Broccoli

All brassica vegetables (think cauliflower, cabbage, kale) have cancer-fighting ingredients, but broccoli is the only one without a hefty portion of sulforaphane, a highly potent component that increases the body's preventive enzymes and washes out chemicals that can cause cancer.

Helps fight: breast, liver, lung, prostate, skin, stomach, and bladder cancers.

Your Rx: The more broccoli, the better the research suggests, so insert it wherever you can, from salads to omelets to the pizza top.

Berries

All the berries are packed with micronutrients which battle against cancer. But black raspberries in particular contain high levels quantities of phytochemicals called anthocyanins, which slow the progression of premalignant cells and preserve new blood cells from establishing and potentially feeding a cancerous tumor.

Helps fight: Colon, esophageal, oral, and skin cancers.

Your Rx: Half a cup of berries a day can also improve your health.

Tomatoes

This juicy fruit is the major diet source of lycopene, a carotenoid that delivers its red hue to tomatoes. And that's great news, because in a research in Nutrition and Cancer, lycopene was found to stop endometrial cancer cell growth. Endometrial cancer kills close to 8,000 people a year.

Helps fight: Endometrial, lung, prostate, and stomach cancers.

Your Rx: The greatest advantage comes from roasted tomatoes (think pasta sauce!), as the heat treatment increases the level of lycopene your body can absorb.

Walnuts

Their phytosterols (cholesterol-like molecules found in plants) have been shown to limit neurons of estrogen in breast cancer cells, potentially slowing the growth of cells.

Helps fight: Breast and prostate cancers

Your Rx: Having a drink 1 ounce of walnuts per day can deliver the best advantages.

Garlic

Phytochemicals in garlic were found to stop nitrosamine formation, carcinogens developed in the stomach (and in the intestines, under certain conditions) when you ingest nitrates, a commonly consumed preservative, Béliveau says. In fact, the Iowa Women's Health researchers showed that women with the highest quantities of garlic in their diets had a 50 percent lower risk of certain colon cancer than those females who took least.

Helps fight: breast, colon, esophageal, and stomach cancers.

Your Rx: Cut a fresh, crushed garlic clove (crushing helps release beneficial enzymes) and squirt it in a tomato sauce that is rich in lycopene while simmering.

Beans

A research performed by Michigan State University found that black and navy beans considerably reduced the incidence of colon cancer in rats, partly because a diet rich in legumes continued to increase fatty acid butyrate levels, which have beneficial effects against cancer growth in high concentrations. The research found that canned beans were especially helpful in preventing breast cancer in rats in the paper Crop

Science.

Helps fight: breast and colon cancers

Your Rx: Attach a serving of legumes few more days per week (from either a can or dry beans that were washed and roasted) to your daily green or other vegetables routine.

What not to eat: Animal fats

While scientists are still trying to find out which foods get the most cancer-preventing benefits, we know what not to eat if you'd like to keep yourself safe.

Animal fats: Meat, cheese, and butter may be rich in saturated fat that has been linked to obesity — a large predictor of cancer. Opt for leaner sources of protein like fish, low-fat dairy and those good-for-you beans.

What not to eat: Processed meats

A right ballpark hot dog or a couple of slices of bacon will not kill you once in a while, but just don't make them a mainstay of your dict. Many steaks tend to have high number of nitrites and nitrates, preservatives that may potentially increase your risk of significant quantities of gastrointestinal and other cancers.

What not to drink: Excessive alcohol

Hold on after a drink! Too much tipping is linked to an increased risk of mouth, esophagus and breast cancers.

www.ingramcontent.com/pod-product-compliance
Lightning Source LLC
Chambersburg PA
CBHW071358210526
45465CB00001B/158